CONCISE GUIDE TO

Clinical Psychiatry

American Psychiatric Press

CONCISE GUIDES

Robert E. Hales, M.D.
Series Editor

Eve Nelson Shapiro
Project Editor

CONCISE GUIDE TO

Clinical Psychiatry

Steven L. Dubovsky, M.D.

Associate Professor of Psychiatry and Medicine
Vice Chairman, Department of Psychiatry
University of Colorado School of Medicine
Denver, Colorado

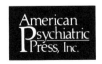

1400 K Street, N.W.
Washington, DC 20005

The paper used in this publication meets the minimum require-
ments of American National Standard for Information Sciences
—Permanence of Paper for Printed Library Materials, ANSI
Z39.48-1984.   ∞

Library of Congress Cataloging-in-Publication Data
Dubovsky, Steven L.
    Concise guide to clinical psychiatry / Steven L. Dubovsky.
— 1st ed.
        p.   cm. — (Concise guides / American Psychiatric
Press)
    Includes bibliographies and index.
    ISBN 0-88048-331-8 (alk. paper)
    1. Psychiatry.   2. Psychotherapy.   I. Title
    II. Series: Concise guides (American Psychiatric Press)
    [DNLM: 1. Mental Disorders.   2. Psychiatry.
    WM 100 D818cb]
RC480.D82 1988
616.89—dc19
DNLM/DLC
for Library of Congress   88-3385
                                                          CIP

To My Family

CONTENTS

Introduction to Concise Guides xi
Preface. xiii
Introduction: *DSM-III-R* xv

1. DEPRESSION **1**
Signs and Symptoms 1
Categories of Depression 4
Present Illness 6
Past History 7
Family History 8
Associated Problems 8
Laboratory Findings. 12
Subtle Presentations of Depression 14
Course 17
Etiology 17
Differential Diagnosis. 21
Treatment. 27
New Nonpharmacologic Physical Treatments
   for Depression. 43
What to Say to Depressed Patients 44
References 47

2. ANXIETY **49**
Anxiety and Fear 50
Signs and Symptoms 50
Categories of Anxiety. 51
Present Illness 55
Past History 56
Family History 56
Associated Problems 57
Laboratory Findings. 59
Course 60
Etiology 60
Differential Diagnosis. 62

Treatment 64

Psychological and Behavioral Management of
Anxious Patients 71

What If the Patient Does Not Respond? 75

References 76

3. SLEEP DISORDERS 77

Signs and Symptoms 78

Categories of Sleep Disorders 79

Present Illness 82

Family History 84

Associated Problems 84

Laboratory Findings 85

Etiology 86

Differential Diagnosis 88

Treatment 90

References 96

**4. SOMATIZATION AND SOMATOFORM
DISORDERS 97**

Signs and Symptoms 97

Categories of Somatoform Disorders 99

Present Illness 101

Past History 101

Family History 101

Associated Problems 102

Laboratory Findings 103

Course 103

Etiology 103

Differential Diagnosis 106

Treatment 109

Management 111

References 113

5. ORGANIC MENTAL SYNDROMES 114

Signs and Symptoms 117

Categories of Organic Mental Syndromes 120

Present Illness 122
Past History 123
Family History 123
Associated Problems 123
Laboratory Findings 124
Subtle Presentations of Dementia 126
Course 126
Etiology 127
Differential Diagnosis 128
Treatment 130
References 136

6. SUBSTANCE ABUSE AND DEPENDENCE . . 138
Definitions 138
Signs and Symptoms 140
Categories of Dependence and Abuse 141
Present Illness and Past History 141
Family History 145
Associated Problems 145
Laboratory Findings 149
Subtle Presentations of Substance Dependence
    and Abuse 150
Course 150
Etiology 151
Differential Diagnosis 152
Treatment 153
Addicted Physicians 161
References 162

7. PSYCHOSIS 164
Signs and Symptoms 164
Categories of Psychosis 167
History 170
Associated Problems 171
Laboratory Findings 175
Course 176
Etiology 176

Differential Diagnosis. 177
Treatment. 179
References 191
Index **193**

INTRODUCTION

to the American Psychiatric Press Concise Guides

The *American Psychiatric Press Concise Guides* series provides, in a most accessible format, practical information for psychiatrists—and especially for psychiatry residents and medical students—working in such varied treatment settings as inpatient psychiatry services, outpatient clinics, consultation/liaison services, and private practice. The *Concise Guides* are meant to complement the more detailed information to be found in lengthier psychiatry texts.

The *Concise Guides* address topics of greatest concern to psychiatrists in clinical practice. The books in this series contain a detailed Table of Contents, along with an index, tables, and charts, for easy access; and their size, designed to fit into a lab coat pocket, makes them a convenient source of information. The number of references has been limited to those most relevant to the material presented.

The *Concise Guide to Clinical Psychiatry*, by Steven L. Dubovsky, M.D., summarizes general clinical psychiatry for medical students who rotate on the psychiatry service during their third-year clerkship, as well as for the psychiatry resident and busy practitioner. Dr. Dubovsky, a noted teacher, skilled clinician, and respected academician, has written several successful psychiatry textbooks. In this book he provides medical students, residents, and staff psychiatrists with a brief overview of the field, presenting practical and clinically useful information with a focus on diagnosis and treatment.

Because these guides are concise, only a select number of topics can be covered. Dr. Dubovsky focuses on those psychiatric disorders encountered most frequently in the general hospital setting: depression, anxiety, sleep disorders, somatoform disorders, organic mental disorders, substance abuse and dependence, and psychosis. Each chapter is structured around the logical examination of the following characteristics of each disorder: epidemiology, signs and symptoms, categories, present illness, past history, family history, associated problems and laboratory findings, course, etiology, differential diagnosis, and treatment.

Consequently, the reader will be able to compare factors among various disorders.

One of the greatest challenges for an author is to be concise. Dr. Dubovsky has succeeded in making the *Concise Guide to Clinical Psychiatry* a useful supplement to major psychiatry texts. It is succinct, easy to read and to use, and provides timely, clinical pearls.

Robert E. Hales, M.D.
Series Editor
American Psychiatric Press Concise Guides

PREFACE

This is the most exciting time in the history of psychiatry. Every day, new discoveries are made that broaden our understanding of the functions and malfunctions of the mind and body and that facilitate clinical management of patients whose problems used to be thought too complicated to handle.

One of the most important advances in recent years has been the acceptance by practitioners in all medical fields that mental phenomena have physical underpinnings, and that physical disorders are affected by mental orientation. Experienced clinicians know that it is impossible to treat a medical disorder effectively without taking into account the patient's emotions, attitudes, and experiences, and it is irresponsible to treat many mental symptoms without at least considering biological interventions. Because the major psychiatric syndromes so clearly manifest themselves in both the psychological and physiological realms, it is particularly easy to apply knowledge of biology and psychology to their management.

This book is a practical guide to the application of modern principles to the psychological and biological treatment of the psychiatric disorders that are most commonly encountered in everyday practice. It is designed for students and residents who wish a comprehensive introduction to the kinds of problems they are likely to encounter on the wards and in the clinics without a detailed examination of every conceivable syndrome and fact. Enough information is provided to carry the reader into practice, where this *Concise Guide to Clinical Psychiatry* can serve as a reminder of important clinical points and a supplement to more detailed texts. The focus is on clinically useful points rather than on theory.

I have tried to focus on approaches to diagnosis and treatment that have been useful in my own and my colleague's work and in the literature in treating real patients in the real world of medicine and psychiatry. Those interested in psychiatry should find material to ground them in essential principles and whet their appetites for more. Those who plan to enter other specialties will find enough information to organize an approach to the psychiatric problems that permeate even the most specialized practice.

Only one word of caution is necessary: As in all other medical specialties, knowledge in psychiatry is accumulating so rapidly that it is necessary for any practitioner to remain continually updated about major new developments. The basic principles outlined in this book are likely to be enduring, but new psychotherapies, new medications, and even new diagnoses are likely to emerge in the next few years. The reader should therefore be prepared to add new information to the foundation that is laid here as well as to consider differing views on the use of available therapies that abound in any rapidly expanding field. Because misprints may occur and differences of opinion may exist, it is important to recheck the dosage and use of any medication before administering it.

Steven L. Dubovsky, M.D.
Denver, Colorado
1988

INTRODUCTION
DSM-III-R

The cornerstone of modern psychiatric diagnosis is the *Diagnostic and Statistical Manual of Mental Disorders, Third Edition, Revised (DSM-III-R)*, which was published by the American Psychiatric Association in 1987 (1). This manual represents a consensus of mental health professionals from a number of disciplines about signs and symptoms that characterize various psychiatric disorders. Making a psychiatric diagnosis with the criteria contained in *DSM-III-R* requires a basic knowledge of its purpose and scope.

DSM-III-R and its predecessor, *DSM-III*, are departures from previous diagnostic schemes in psychiatry in that they attempt to be as atheoretical as possible in their orientation. Psychiatric conditions are referred to as disorders rather than diseases in order to avoid implying etiologies about which reasonable disagreement might exist, which would get in the way of using the diagnosis clinically. This does not mean that the *DSM-III-R* disorders do not have etiologies; it just means that the formal diagnostic nomenclature is concerned only with signs, symptoms, and course.

The second important point about *DSM-III-R* is that it is multiaxial; that is, it assesses patients with respect to several dimensions at the same time. The purpose of this method of classification is to force clinicians to consider psychiatric disturbances on more than one level. A diagnosis on one axis does not restrict diagnoses on other axes, and several diagnoses may coexist at the same time on any axis.

Axis I (clinical syndromes) includes disorders that are departures from a person's usual level of functioning. The implication of an Axis I diagnosis is that if the clinician looks carefully enough, the disorder can often be seen to have its onset at some specific point and to vary over time, although in some cases it can be difficult, if not impossible, to differentiate such disorders from the presumably more stable disturbances of personality that are diagnosed on Axis II.

Axis II is used for diagnosing personality disorders, which

are enduring constellations of inflexible, maladaptive behaviors and traits that are manifest by adolescence or early adulthood, and that cause subjective distress and/or impair social or occupational functioning. Developmental disorders, or pervasive impairments that begin in childhood such as mental retardation, autism, and dyslexia, are also diagnosed on Axis II. Axis I diagnoses are used throughout this book. Where appropriate, personality disorders are mentioned; but because they are a more specialized topic they are not described in detail. Instead, they will be introduced very briefly here. Advanced reviews can be found in the references at the end of this section (2,3).

■ PERSONALITY DISORDERS

Antisocial personality disorder has been the most carefully studied of the Axis II diagnoses. This disorder is characterized by various kinds of antisocial behavior such as truancy, violence, stealing, and lying beginning before the age of 15. Patients with antisocial behavior are disloyal, aggressive, untrustworthy, untruthful, impulsive, irresponsible and reckless, with poor judgment and inability to function reliably at work or at home. A personality disorder that is grouped with antisocial personality in the "dramatic" cluster of personality disorders in *DSM-III-R* is *borderline personality disorder*. This personality disorder is characterized by unstable emotions and relationships, impulsive and manipulative self-destructive behavior, angry outbursts, identity disturbances, and severe fears of abandonment. *Narcissistic personality disorder* is related psychologically to borderline personality. The principle manifestations of narcissistic personality described by *DSM-III-R* concern unrealistic grandiosity, chronic envy, exploitativeness, lack of empathy, endless need for admiration and attention, and a sense of being entitled to special favors without having to earn them.

A second cluster of personality disorders includes those characterized by extreme social discomfort and fears of being embarrassed or hurt, which lead to avoidance unless the patient is certain of being liked *(avoidant personality disorder)*; dependency, submissiveness, and preoccupation with not being alone *(dependent personality disorder)*; perfectionism, inflexibility, indecisiveness, overconscientiousness, having to have one's own way, being undemonstrative and ungenerous and preoccupation with rules and details *(obsessive compulsive personality disorder)*; and expression of hostility through passive resistance in the form of procrastination, forgetting obligations, complaining that too much is being demanded, and working too slowly or doing a bad job *(passive-aggressive personality disorder)*.

A third cluster of personality disorders as defined in *DSM-III-R* consists of syndromes of odd interactions with others. *Paranoid personality disorder* is characterized by a view of the world as dangerous or demeaning, so that the patient is habitually jealous, easily slighted, resentful, secretive, and suspicious. In *schizoid personality disorder*, the patient seems to have no interest in forming relationships and little ability to express emotions. *Schizotypal personality disorder* probably is related to schizophrenia. It is characterized by stable traits that are not quite psychotic but may later deteriorate into a schizophrenic psychosis. Examples include the patient's feeling but not being certain that people are talking about him or her, magical beliefs, sensing but not actually seeing things or people that are not actually there, eccentric behavior, vague, abstract speech, silly or aloof emotional expression, and excessive suspiciousness.

Axis III in *DSM-III-R* is for physical conditions that may be affecting psychiatric symptoms. Axis IV contains a scale for judging the severity of stresses ranging from mild to catastrophic that may be contributing to an Axis I disorder. Axis V consists of an instrument for formally rating a patient's overall level of functioning.

DSM-III-R criteria are used throughout this book. Additional diagnostic clues are added when appropriate, and physical and psychological causes that are not included in the nomenclature are considered where appropriate.

■ REFERENCES

1. American Psychiatric Association: Diagnostic and Statistical Manual of Mental Disorders, 3rd edition, revised. Washington DC, American Psychiatric Association, 1987
2. Reid WH (Ed): The Treatment of Antisocial Syndromes. New York, Van Nostrand Reinhold, 1981
3. Kernberg OF: Borderline Conditions and Pathological Narcissism. New York, Jason Aronson, 1975

DEPRESSION 1

Depression is one of the most common conditions encountered by physicians. At any given time, 9–20% of all people have at least some significant depressive symptoms and 4–6% have the full-blown clinical picture of depression. For unknown reasons, women become depressed twice as frequently as men. Of everyone reading this book, 8–9% will be clearly depressed at some point in their lives and another 2–4% will have more subtle forms of depression. This means that more than 10% of the population—more than 30 million individuals in the United States alone—are vulnerable to depression (1).

In all industrialized countries of the world, the incidence of depression has been increasing with each decade since 1910. The chance of getting depressed has increased and the age at which depression first appears has decreased in every generation born after World War II. It is not that people are recognizing depression or seeking treatment earlier; for some unknown reason more people are actually becoming depressed, and they are doing so at a younger age.

Less than one-fourth of the millions of people who become depressed receive any treatment at all. One reason for this state of affairs is that many depressed individuals believe that it is weak, sick, or humiliating to ask for help and so they suffer alone. If they do reveal their distress, it is frequently in the form of physical symptoms, which feel more acceptable than emotional complaints. Another reason for the massive undertreatment of depression is that many physicians dismiss it as a normal or expectable reaction to life stress that does not require specific care. But depression is a distinct pathological entity with many differences from what Freud referred to as "the misery of everyday life."

■ SIGNS AND SYMPTOMS

Everyone has depressive feelings from time to time, especially at times of loss, disappointment, and change. Normally, such feelings are short-lived and do not interfere with everyday functioning. A little reassurance, a display of affection from a loved one, or a change of scene helps, and even if the situation that evokes unhappiness does not change it is usually possible to adapt.

Depression, on the other hand, is a more pervasive and enduring experience. Depressed affect (emotional expression), which extends beyond simple sadness, is accompanied by disturbances of thinking, behavior, and biological function that become more or less autonomous from whatever experiences may have initiated them. Depression as a clinical syndrome is diagnosed when a cluster of specific dysfunctions in each of these psychobiological spheres is identified.

MOOD

The mood (enduring emotional tone) of someone who is depressed is typically sad, tearful, unhappy, and discouraged. Irritability, hostility, or feelings of emptiness, apathy, and lack of motivation may overshadow depressive mood, particularly in depressed children and adolescents and in chronically depressed adults. Anxiety accompanies depression in 70–80% of cases, and 20% develop full-blown panic attacks (1). The earliest emotional clue to depression may be anhedonia, or loss of the capacity to experience pleasure, humor, or happiness.

THINKING

Negative thinking is a hallmark of depression. People who are depressed generalize from one experience (e.g., "my children didn't pay attention to me when I came home from work") to more global negative conclusions (e.g., "nobody loves me"). They then ignore evidence that contradicts negative assumptions about themselves, other people, and the future and overemphasize minor setbacks that seem to prove their beliefs. Believing that nothing will change, the depressed person makes no attempt to improve a bad situation. As a result nothing changes, and the belief that the situation is hopeless is reinforced.

A fundamentally negative orientation toward oneself in depression can be manifested as self-blame for everything that goes wrong while feeling incapable of doing anything right. Even if they thought that it were possible to feel better, depressed patients may feel that they do not deserve to improve. This heightened sense of guilt and unworthiness, combined with negative thinking about the future, makes death seem appealing as a deserved punishment and as the only way to exert control over one's life.

Depression slows thinking, making it difficult to concentrate and remember. These disturbances are probably not just due to preoccupation with unhappiness and psychological problems but may also reflect changes in brain function. In fact, many clinicians find it difficult if not impossible to differentiate between the cognitive dysfunction of depression and that of organic brain disease, especially in the elderly.

BEHAVIOR

Depressed people frequently become dependent, passive, and helpless, at times covertly using their symptoms to manipulate others into meeting their needs. Paradoxically, however, when others attempt to help, their offers of assistance are refused. The reason for this apparent contradiction is that the depressed person feels insecure and needy but is also humiliated by even normal needs and is hostile toward anyone who, by being able to provide support, reminds the patient of needs that the patient despises. At the same time, the depressed patient, who usually has had previous unresolved experiences with loss, is exquisitely sensitive to rejection.

Problems in important relationships frequently lead to marital discord and trouble on the job. Feeling incapable of functioning socially, the depressed individual begins to avoid interacting with others, which only increases feelings of loneliness and rejection. The patient may yearn for contact, but on the surface is hostile and withdrawn in order to keep at a distance those who might hurt the patient by abandonment. Covert forms of self-destructive behavior, such as accident proneness and alienating friends and superiors at work, are common in chronically depressed individuals.

BIOLOGICAL FUNCTIONS

Depression produces numerous important alterations of basic vegetative function. The most common abnormality is disturbed sleep. Most depressed patients have difficulty falling and staying asleep; 20–30% sleep too much. Appetite and weight can be increased or decreased. The overall level of energy and activity is frequently decreased, although the patient may also engage in endless futile agitation. Constipation, impotence, and various physical complaints are also common somatic manifestations of depression.

Frequently there is an endogenous rhythm to depressed mood so that it is characteristically worse in the morning (diurnal rhythm) or evening (reverse diurnal rhythm). Depression also may have an annual rhythm that makes it worse at one time of year (usually but not always the winter) than another. In women, hormonal rhythms may make depression worse in association with the menstrual cycle, pregnancy, or childbirth.

■ CATEGORIES OF DEPRESSION

Depression can be classified in a number of ways. Common diagnostic categories include:

MAJOR DEPRESSION

This is the term used in the current nomenclature to indicate a typical depressive episode that has been present for at least two weeks and is characterized by the daily presence of at least five common disturbances, one of which must be a change in mood or the ability to experience pleasure. Signs and symptoms of major depression may include a pervasive depressed or irritable mood, diminished interest or pleasure in usual activities, appetite and/or weight change, sleep disturbance, psychomotor agitation or retardation, fatigue or loss of energy, feelings of worthlessness or guilt, decreased concentration, and recurrent thoughts of death or suicide.

MAJOR DEPRESSION, MELANCHOLIC TYPE (ENDOGENOUS DEPRESSION)

The term endogenous depression usually is used to indicate that depression is accompanied by vegetative changes or other signs of a prominent disturbance of biological function. Endogenous depression tends to be more severe, and the patient is not at all cheered by positive events or by other people. Depression with melancholic (endogenous) features is more likely to respond to physical interventions. Whether or not there has been a clearcut psychosocial precipitant of depression is *not* correlated with the degree to which melancholia is present.

MAJOR DEPRESSION WITH PSYCHOTIC FEATURES (PSYCHOTIC DEPRESSION)

In about 10% of cases (25% of depressed inpatients), depression is accompanied by symptoms of psychosis (delusions, hallucinations, loss of reality testing). Psychotic symptoms in depression are usually but not always consistent with a depressed mood (e.g., delusions of being punished by having a terrible disease or hallucinated voices telling the patient to commit suicide). The risk of suicide is five to six times higher in psychotic depression.

DYSTHYMIA (CHRONIC DEPRESSION)

Chronic low grade depression that has been present for at least two years (one year in children and adolescents) but has not been of sufficient severity to warrant a diagnosis of major depression is called dysthymia in the current nomenclature. The relationship of more subtle forms of depression to major depression is discussed below.

PRIMARY DEPRESSION

When depression occurs by itself, it is said to be primary. The term secondary depression is used to refer to depression that occurs in the context of another psychiatric, medical, or surgical condition (e.g., depression in a schizophrenic). This is not an official term but it is used by many investigators to differentiate conditions in which depression is the only problem from those in which it may interact with other disorders.

BIPOLAR DISORDER

In bipolar disorder (manic depressive illness), the patient has experienced at least one episode of mania or hypomania (see below). At any one time, bipolar depression may be predominantly manic, depressed, or mixed (i.e., manic and depressive symptoms occur at the same time).

SEASONAL AFFECTIVE DISORDER (SADs)

SADs is an annual rhythm of depression in which depression occurs in the fall and winter, sometimes accompanied by hypomania in the spring (2). SADs appears to be caused by seasonal variations in light and can be cured or prevented by bright light of the intensity of sunlight. In reverse SADs, depression occurs in the summer and hypomania may occur in the winter.

■ PRESENT ILLNESS

Certain experiences or emotions commonly lead to depression. The diagnosis should be considered when a patient develops psychiatric symptoms in the context of one of these situations (3, 4).

LOSS

Depression frequently appears following a loss. The loss may be of a person, health, financial status, control, or attention from others. The loss may be real, or it may be threatened or imagined. A trivial loss to one person may be devastating to another. People can be sensitized to react to loss with depression if they:

- did not expect the loss
- have experienced previous losses
- had strongly mixed feelings about the person who was lost
- are excessively dependent on a lost person, ideal, thing, or quality for self-esteem, security, or a sense of inner intactness
- cannot tolerate the grief that normally follows a loss
- have been depressed in the past
- have a family history of depression.

INTERPERSONAL PROBLEMS

Even if actual loss is not an issue, problems in an ongoing relationship may lead to depression. Disputes about marital roles, important transitions such as from active work to retirement, and feelings of being unable to influence the partner, express anger, or be independent are common settings in which depression develops. Many of these problems become self-perpetuating when the depressed person becomes irritable, dependent, and sensitive to rejection, alienating others before they have a chance to leave of their own accord.

HELPLESSNESS

Any situation that evokes feelings of helplessness and passivity can lead to depression. This is a common problem for patients with chronic medical illnesses who feel that the disease process is out of their control. They cannot make themselves better, but they may be able to achieve some sense of control by making things worse through noncompliance, active aggravation of the illness, or by frustrating doctors and nurses, making them feel more helpless than the patient.

■ PAST HISTORY

Frequently depression is chronic or recurrent. A current episode may be a continuation of an incompletely resolved previous episode requiring a change in treatment, or a new recurrence that will respond to the same treatment again. The presence of manic symptoms in the past also may alter treatment decisions in the present. It is therefore important to assess:

- *Number and course of previous episodes:* Depression tends to become more severe and complex with age; is this episode significantly different from previous ones?
- *Completeness of remission of previous episodes:* Relapse is more likely if an episode of depression has not completely remitted.
- *Past history of treatment for depression:* What has helped and what has not? Treatments that have been successful in the past are more likely to be effective again.
- *Past history of mania:* Patients who have been manic (see below) may follow a different course and require different therapeutic strategies than those who only have been depressed.

■ FAMILY HISTORY

The rate of depression is at least twice as high in the first degree relatives of depressed patients than in the general population. People with familial loading for depression tend to become depressed earlier in life and to have a greater number of recurrences than those who have fewer depressed relatives. A family history of mania increases the likelihood that a patient will become manic as well as depressed (5).

Suicide, alcoholism, and/or antisocial behavior also tend to cluster in the families of some depressed patients. A family history of any of these conditions, as well as of depression and mania, therefore increases the likelihood that a patient with an unclear illness is depressed. The response of family members to treatments for depression can be helpful in guiding treatment selection for a patient because inherited patterns of metabolism of antidepressants may predict a response to a treatment that has been helpful to a blood relative.

The familial transmission of depression and related conditions has been the subject of a good deal of study. Depressed people may function poorly as parents if they continually threaten abandonment, openly express hostility, belittle their children, or are too withdrawn to be emotionally available. This kind of parenting causes emotional problems in the children, but it may not of necessity lead only to depression. Adoption and twin studies suggest a genetic component that makes blood relatives of depressives vulnerable to develop depression instead of some other disorder. Recent investigations have actually identified genetic markers for bipolar disorder that suggest a single locus on chromosome #11 in one population of Amish subjects and on the x-chromosome in several Middle Eastern families. The inheritance of the propensity to depression without mania is thought to be polygenic.

■ ASSOCIATED PROBLEMS

Depression may be associated with several psychiatric disorders that significantly affect its course, prognosis, and treatment. The routine evaluation of any depressed patient should include assessments for these conditions.

MANIA

Phenomenologically, mania appears to be the opposite of depression. However, in many ways there are more similarities than differences between the two states. Biological abnormalities in both are similar if not identical, both run in the same families, and depression frequently alternates or is mixed with mania. About 30% of depressives are subject to bouts of mania, while the vast majority of manics eventually become depressed.

Typical manic symptoms include heightened level of activity, effort, and sexual interest, grandiosity, rapid, pressured, speech, increased energy, decreased need for sleep, distractibility, and poor judgment that usually involves overestimation of the patient's abilities and resources. Depression that is complicated at some point in its course by mania is called *bipolar disorder*. People who only become depressed are said to have *unipolar depression*. One important treatment implication of this distinction is that patients with bipolar disorder are subject to both mania and increased depressive relapses if they are treated incautiously with antidepressants.

When manic symptoms are not sufficiently severe to be grossly disabling, they are referred to collectively as *hypomania*. If a bipolar disorder is associated with full-blown mania, it is called bipolar I disorder. If only hypomania is experienced, the disorder is bipolar II. Although patients with mania (i.e., bipolar disorder I) may also experience hypomania, there is a group of patients with hypomania (bipolar II disorder) who never become manic. Patients with bipolar II disorder tend to have relatives with bipolar II but not bipolar I disorder and vice versa, suggesting that the two conditions are genetically distinct. From a clinical standpoint, bipolar II disorder appears to be intermediate in severity between bipolar I disorder and unipolar depression.

SUBSTANCE ABUSE

Abuse of central nervous system (CNS) depressants such as alcohol and tranquilizers is common in depressed patients. The sedative effect of these substances temporarily relieves distress and insomnia, but in the long run they actually increase depression. Alcohol and barbiturates also increase hepatic breakdown of antidepressants, adding metabolic antagonism to the central antagonism of the effect of the antidepressant.

All depressed patients should be questioned carefully about their use of centrally acting substances. There is little point in attempting to treat depression without first addressing continued intake of these drugs, because their pharmacological effects aggravate depression and interfere with response to antidepressants, and because the patient who refuses to attempt to discontinue them is expressing, at best, ambivalent motivation to improve.

SUICIDE

Suicide is a complication of up to 15% of cases of depression. Many demographic factors (e.g., being older, being male, experiencing social isolation, or having chronic or terminal illness) have been said to increase the risk. The most clinically meaningful risk factors include (6, 7):

Past history of suicide attempts. The ultimate risk of suicide may be lower in patients who repeatedly make minor manipulative suicide attempts as opposed to those who have made dangerous attempts in which rescue was unlikely. However, this often is a difficult clinical distinction, and anyone who has made two or more attempts should be considered at significant risk. The danger of suicide if the patient becomes depressed again is particularly high if previous attempts have been violent and premeditated.

Expression of hopelessness. People contemplate suicide because they feel that they have no other option to end suffering, influence others, or resolve feelings about a loved one who has died. Patients who feel hopeless about their depression, or about the chances of recovering from a physical illness or solving an important problem, are at increased risk of suicide.

Anxiety. Severe anxiety in a depressed patient may increase the risk of suicide, perhaps because it indicates a more severe episode of depression.

Family history of suicide. Family members who have committed suicide have transmitted a genetic vulnerability and have served as role models for suicide as an acceptable means of problem solving.

Presence of a viable plan. The greatest risk is in people who have a concrete suicide plan that can be carried out in the near future (e.g., a patient who wants to shoot himself who has a loaded gun at home), especially if they have rehearsed the plan (e.g., putting an empty gun to their head and pulling the trigger) and if nothing prevents them from carrying it out. Those who describe unrealistic plans (e.g., swimming out to sea when there is no ocean nearby) and those with powerful reasons not to die (e.g., religious beliefs or for the sake of the children) are at less risk but may become more dangerous if they suffer a setback or deteriorate emotionally. Patients with suicidal thoughts but no plans are usually not high risks, but their ideas need to be reevaluated regularly to ensure that they have not become more dangerous to themselves.

Diagnosis of depression and/or alcoholism. Suicide occurs most frequently in patients who are depressed (especially bipolar I disorder, and severe and psychotic depression) and alcoholic. Patients with schizophrenia, narcotic abuse, and organic brain disease also kill themselves at a higher rate than the general population. Character disorders and other psychiatric diagnoses are not predictably associated with an increased rate of suicide.

Encouragement of suicide by significant others. Family members and friends may covertly encourage a patient to commit suicide, or at least may not be aggressive in discouraging the idea when the patient has been chronically depressed or suicidal, when the patient is hostile and provocative, when significant conflict existed before the patient became depressed, or when the significant other is depressed too. An effective management plan must include other important people in such cases if suicide is to be prevented.

Communication of intent. Of all people who kill themselves, at least two-thirds tell a family member, friend, or physician about their intent. It is therefore a fatal mistake to believe the popular myth that people who talk about suicide do not act on their ideas.

DEPRESSION IN FAMILY AND FRIENDS

Like most people with similar traits, depressed individuals tend to marry each other at a rate that is higher than would be expected by chance (assortative mating). For this reason, depressed patients often have depressed spouses. If the spouses do not wish to think of themselves as depressed, they may encourage the patient to display serious symptoms in order to keep the focus of treatment on the patient and away from their own problems. At the same time, they may vicariously receive treatment through the patient's therapy.

Even when the spouse is not depressed to begin with, marital discord is a common problem that is produced by the depressed patient's hostility, withdrawal, and inability to experience pleasure. Fears of rejection may lead some depressed patients to provoke their partners into leaving so that the patient will not have to wait passively to be abandoned. Genetic transmission of vulnerability to depression and the effects of depression on parenting skills increase the likelihood of behavior and school problems, substance abuse, medical illness, and depression in the children of depressed patients.

NONCOMPLIANCE

The negative thinking of depression makes noncompliance a frequent complication because the patient does not believe that treatment will help or does not feel entitled to get better. When such patients remain depressed they conclude that they were right all along not to trust the therapy, ignoring the fact that their failure to improve is due to their own behavior and not the inadequacy of the treatment. Some patients who have become accustomed to a depressive lifestyle may discontinue a useful therapy when they feel threatened by the possibility of feeling well. Covert noncompliance and inadequate motivation for self-care are common causes of apparent resistance to medically adequate therapy in depressed physically ill patients.

■ LABORATORY FINDINGS

Abnormalities in several laboratory tests have been reported in depression. The significant number of false negatives and false positives, especially in a medically ill population, makes these tests unsuitable for routine screening for depression (8). However, in selected cases, certain tests can be helpful in clarifying the diagnosis, following treatment response, and convincing patients that they have a "real" problem. From a conceptual standpoint, they demonstrate that depression has a biological as well as a psychological component.

DEXAMETHASONE SUPPRESSION TEST

About 50% of depressed patients fail to suppress serum cortisol on the day after administration of dexamethasone (9). This phenomenon is measured with the dexamethasone suppression test (DST), which is performed by administering 1 mg of dexamethasone orally at 11 PM and determining serum cortisol levels the next day at 4 PM for outpatients, and at 8 AM, 4 PM, and 11 PM for inpatients. In most laboratories, a serum cortisol on any determination greater than 5 μg/dl indicates nonsuppression. Severe acute stress, recent hospitalization, weight loss, pregnancy, temporal lobe epilepsy, various endocrinopathies, and medications or drugs that increase the metabolism of dexamethasone can produce apparent nonsuppression in patients who are not depressed (8). In the absence of any confounding factors, DST nonsuppression strongly suggests depression. A normal DST is of no diagnostic significance.

When it happens to be positive, the DST often reverts to normal suppression shortly before clinical improvement. Nonsuppression may reappear in advance of reappearance of depressive symptoms. If the DST remains nonsuppressed in a patient who has responded to an antidepressant, depression is more likely to return if the medication is withdrawn than if the DST has normalized. A persistently positive DST therefore suggests that antidepressant therapy should be continued (10).

THYROTROPIN RELEASING HORMONE STIMULATION TEST

Roughly one-third of depressed patients (not necessarily the same ones with a nonsuppressed DST) demonstrate a subnormal (blunted) rise in thyroid-stimulating hormone (TSH) following the intravenous infusion of 500 μg of thyrotropin releasing hormone (TRH) (11). The TRH stimulation test is not a practical office test for depression, but it does indicate that activation of the hypothalamic-pituitary-thyroid axis accompanies the activation of the hypothalamic-pituitary-adrenal axis that is indicated by nonsuppression on the DST. Both abnormalities probably originate at the level of the hypothalamus or above.

SLEEP EEG

As many as 80% of depressed patients exhibit early appearance after sleep onset of the first rapid eye movement (REM) period (decreased REM latency) on a sleep electroencephalogram (EEG). Other sleep abnormalities that have been reported in depression include a shift of more REM sleep to the first half of the night, allowing less time for the slow wave sleep that normally occurs at this time, and increased eye movements when REM sleep occurs (increased REM density). Some authorities question the specificity of sleep EEG abnormalities for depression, but many consider the sleep EEG a reliable test when it is properly performed (12).

■ SUBTLE PRESENTATIONS OF DEPRESSION

A change in mood is the hallmark of depression. However, in as many as 50% of patients encountered in medical practice, emotional symptoms are much less obvious than disturbances of thinking, behavior, social and occupational function that are derivatives of the depressed state of mind (Table 1). Several syndromes of "marked" depression are common.

MULTIPLE SOMATIC COMPLAINTS

Patients who are unable to express emotions in words frequently experience mental pain as a physical disturbance. Unable to tell the difference between their minds and their bodies, these patients consider it weak or disgraceful to be mentally but not physically ill. Instead of feeling unhappy when they become depressed, they develop fatigue, back pain, headaches, insomnia, constipation, or other somatic disturbances.

TABLE 1. **Clues to Covert Depression**

Previous episodes of depression, mania, or response to antidepressant

Family history of depression, mania, suicide, alcoholism or antisocial behavior

Personality change

Substance abuse

Negativism

Marital problems

Frequent job changes

Persistent insomnia

Unexplained physical complaint

Hostility, cynicism, pessimism

Passivity, low self-confidence

Accident proneness

Antisocial behavior or school problems in a teenager

Loss of sense of humor

All-or-nothing thinking

Atypical psychosis

SUBAFFECTIVE PERSONALITY SYNDROMES

When emotional expression is distorted, depression and mania can be transformed into distortions of the personality that reflect depressive and/or manic orientations without clearcut changes in mood. These disturbances are said to be "subsyndromal" or "subaffective" because they are not clearcut enough to meet formal criteria for an affective (depressive or manic) disorder (13). The following three subaffective syndromes have been described.

SUBAFFECTIVE DEPRESSION (DYSTHYMIA)

This is a subtle form of depression that skews character in the direction of easy disappointment, pessimism, insufficient energy to engage in positive tasks, and readiness to retreat. Patients with dysthymia are habitually gloomy, introverted, passive, demanding, negativistic people who fear intimacy at the same time that they crave it. What relationships dysthymic individuals do maintain tend to be pervaded by angry accusations about their own and others' inadequacies, and cynical enjoyment of defeat and unhappiness.

SUBAFFECTIVE MANIA

This is subclinical mania expressed through the personality in the form of such traits as arrogance, insensitivity, talkativeness, emotional intensity, temper tantrums, promiscuity, and unpredictability. Many patients with subaffective mania abuse psychoactive drugs in an attempt to tone down hyperactive emotionality.

CYCLOTHYMIA

This is a subsyndromal variant of bipolar disorder in which manic and depressive traits alternate with each other. Cyclothymic individuals may be withdrawn and insecure some of the time, and hyperactive, hypersexual, irritable, and pushy at other times.

APROSODIAS

Language has two important components that interact to convey the richness of meaning inherent in even the simplest communication. The *propositional* component of language is comprised of various aspects of content such as words, phrases, sentences, grammar, and syntax. Disorders of propositional speech, which result from lesions of the dominant hemisphere (usually the left), are called *aphasias*.

The second major component of language is called *prosody*. Prosody consists of the pauses, intonations, stresses, accents, and melodic qualities of speech that modify the propositional parts to impart nuances, subtleties, differences in emphasis, social meaning, attitudes, and emotional coloring. Gestures, facial expressions, tone of voice, and other nonverbal cues also are important aspects of prosody. Prosody resides mainly in the nondominant hemisphere, and lesions of this side of the brain may produce disorders of emotional language and behavior that are termed *aprosodias* (14). Analagous to aphasias, aprosodias disrupt expression, comprehension, and repetition of complex emotional messages.

Because patients with aprosodia cannot communicate their mood normally, it can be particularly difficult to recognize when they are depressed. Clues to depression in patients with diseases of the brain that could be causing aprosodia include negativism, noncompliance, refusal to eat or drink, hopelessness, oppositional behavior, expression of a wish to die, irritability, and flattened, labile, inappropriate, bizarre, or silly affect. Abnormal integration of a depressed mood with verbal and behavioral systems can produce such dysregulated emotional behaviors as unusual or incoherent speech, temper outbursts, agitation, mutism, withdrawal, psychomotor retardation, and catatonia. Depression should be considered as a cause of any unusual psychiatric syndrome associated with a past or family history of mood disorder or with vegetative symptoms that are not clearly due to a medical illness.

■ COURSE

Of acutely depressed patients, 50–80% have at least one recurrence; most have several. Patients with unipolar depression have an average of four recurrences, while patients with bipolar depression have twice as many episodes. Recurrences tend to become more frequent, more severe, and longer-lasting with age, especially in bipolar patients. Each recurrence repeats symptoms of previous episodes and adds new symptoms.

Without treatment, 50–60% of patients with acute depression remit spontaneously; untreated patients who have not improved within two years are unlikely to do so. Even with appropriate therapy, up to 15% of depressed patients remain ill. The rate of improvement declines substantially after 18 months of appropriate treatment.

■ ETIOLOGY

Like all mental disorders, depression has a biological as well as a psychological dimension. Each influences the other, and treatment directed at one may lead to enduring changes in the other.

BIOLOGICAL FACTORS

Much recent research has focused on deep cerebral alerting, orienting, motivational and behavioral systems that utilize as neurotransmitters biogenic (biologically active) amines (4, 15). Norepinephrine, a transmitter of activating centers, appears to be dysregulated in depression, with excessive bursts of activity in response to minor stresses and inadequate responses to more significant threats. Noradrenergic dysregulation could account in part for inappropriate activation of stress response systems (e.g., excess cortisol levels with loss of normal diurnal variation and resistance to suppression) that characterize even the most withdrawn depressions. Cerebrospinal fluid (CSF) and urine metabolite studies suggest that activity of serotonin in the brain may be more consistently decreased, perhaps accounting for sleep and appetite disturbances and for the reduced capacity for self-soothing of the depressed individual. Acetylcholine, a transmitter in punishment and withdrawal circuits, has been thought to be hyperactive in depression; and dopamine, which along with acetylcholine is important in motor and motivational systems, may also be dysregulated.

The primary dysfunction in brain neurotransmitter systems is thought to reside in receptor mechanisms as much as in the production and release of transmitter. However, since there is extensive communication within the synapse, abnormalities in receptors would be expected to affect transmitter synthesis and vice versa. Because each neuron in the brain connects to 3,000–10,000 other neurons, a change in one transmitter must affect other transmitters as well, and a resetting of only one system is very unlikely to explain depression.

Depression is associated with disruption of important rhythms of biological activity. For example, the sleep cycle may be phase advanced (turned ahead), first producing early onset of sleep and then of awakening with respect to the time of day. A phase advance of the REM sleep cycle with respect to sleep onset explains decreased REM latency (i.e., early onset of REM after sleep begins) in depression. Phase changes and desynchronization of important biological rhythms from each other are thought by some investigators to be a cause rather than a manifestation of depression. In favor of this hypothesis is the observation that artificially resetting some biological rhythms by changing sleep and REM patterns may aggravate or ameliorate mood disorders.

A more basic view of the psychobiology of depression is that it involves a reorientation of subcellular mechanisms that are common to multiple systems of the body (16). When it affects the brain, a basic disturbance in the regulatory processes of the cell could produce mental symptoms and altered biological rhythms. Its action in the body could at the same time lead to changes in hormone activity. Alterations have been observed in such basic intracellular mechanisms as receptor signaling and the action of calcium ions within peripheral cells such as red blood cells, lymphocytes, and blood platelets. If similar changes occur in the brain, depression may truly be a multisystem disorder.

PSYCHOLOGICAL FACTORS

Since experience can alter neuronal function in the directions that have been implicated in depression (15), it is likely that depression can be produced by primary disturbances of physiological homeostasis that affect the orientation of the mind as well as the body, or by intrapsychic or social pressures that affect the orientation of the body as well as the mind.

UNRESOLVED GRIEF

When an important loss is not mourned, sadness, anger, and a sense of being unable to adapt without the lost person or quality may result in the inconsolable unhappiness, irritability, arousal, sensitivity to rejection, hopelessness, and low self-esteem of depression.

UNEXPRESSED ANGER

Some people find it impossible to express anger, disagreement, or independence because they are afraid that the target of these feelings will retaliate by rejecting them or that being angry or even different is incompatible with loving another person. But anger is an inevitable aspect of human experience, especially if one feels so controlled that it seems impossible to express differences of opinion without fearing rejection. By turning anger against oneself in the form of depression, it is possible to inhibit the expression of anger and punish oneself for having feelings that seem unacceptable. The depression that results can then serve as a covert vehicle for expressing anger when it frustrates and confuses the other person.

ALL-OR-NOTHING THINKING

Many depressed people subscribe to basic assumptions (schemata) about themselves and others that paint the world in one-dimensional black and white terms, examples of which are listed in Table 2 (17). When a minor setback disappoints their impossible expectations, they react with a global judgment about themselves (e.g., "I'll never be happy," or "nobody loves me") and a global feeling of hopelessness and depression.

SELF-FULFILLING PROPHECIES

People who expect the worst tend to look for the worst and to make the worst happen. For example, if a man who believes that his illness will never improve does not take care of himself or follow medical advice, the illness will not get better, and his

TABLE 2. **Typical All-or-Nothing Assumptions in Depression**

If something isn't done perfectly it's worthless
If I can't do something exactly right, there's no point in trying
If I can't do everything I can't do anything
If everyone doesn't love me, nobody cares about me at all
Loving someone means you can never be angry at them
If I get anything from anyone I'm totally dependent
If I do anything for myself I have to do everything for myself
If I'm not constantly admired I'm worthless
If I have any flaws at all, I'm riddled with imperfections
If I'm not happy all the time, I'll always be unhappy
If I'm angry at anyone, I don't love them

negative belief will be confirmed. By paying attention to negative information and discounting positive data, depressed people become more and more convinced that their global negative beliefs are true.

LEARNED HELPLESSNESS

One form of negative expectation is helplessness. The belief that nothing can be done on one's own behalf can be induced by remaining for an extended period of time in a situation over which one has no control. Even when the situation changes, the feeling of helplessness may be reinforced through a self-fulfilling prophecy in which the patient believes that nothing will help, does not exert enough effort, fails, and feels even more helpless. Patients who learned when they were younger that important people do not notice or respond to them unless they were really miserable, for example, may use depression as a primary means of communication because they do not know how to influence other people through more positive emotions. They do not learn to assert themselves constructively because, believing that they cannot, they never try.

■ DIFFERENTIAL DIAGNOSIS

Many common illnesses (Table 3), medications (Table 4) and nonprescription drugs (Table 5) can produce depression that is

TABLE 3. Illnesses That May Cause Depression

Viral infections (especially hepatitis and infectious mononucleosis)

Cancers (e.g., pancreatic carcinoma, leukemia)

Endocrine disease (thyroid, parathyroid, adrenal, pituitary)

Collagen disease

Anemia, especially pernicious anemia

Liver disease

Postcardiotomy states

Stroke

Organic brain disease of any kind

TABLE 4. **Medications That May Cause Depression**

Adrenal steroids and ACTH

Amantadine

Asparaginase

Bromocriptine

Carbamazepine — antiseizure med

Cimetidine

Clonazepam

Digitalis

Disulfiram

L-dopa

Methylopa

Metoclopramide

Oral contraceptives

Phenytoin

Propranolol

Reserpine

Spironolactone

Vinblastine

TABLE 5. **Nonprescription Drugs That May Cause Depression**

Amphetamine withdrawal

Alcohol

Cocaine

Narcotics

Sedatives and tranquilizers

indistinguishable from the primary psychiatric disorder. Partial complex seizures, tertiary syphilis, Cushing's syndrome, and a number of medications (Table 6) may produce manic symptoms. Depression and mania caused by illnesses and psychoactive substances (*organic mood syndromes*) are not emotional reactions to the physical condition but are mental states caused by the direct effect of the illness or substance on the brain. Treatment of the illness, discontinuation of the illicit drug, or a change of medication should be undertaken before treating the mood disorder. If the physical disease cannot be cured or a specific drug (e.g., prednisone) is essential, treatment with an antidepressant may still be helpful.

Depression can easily be confused with a number of disorders in addition to organic mood syndromes, including:

Dementia and delirium: Depression may be associated with significant disturbances of attention, concentration, and short-term memory. These intellectual deficits are due in part to being distracted by dysphoric emotions and thoughts and in part to the same neuronal dysregulation that destabilizes emotion. The result may be a syndrome that is clinically difficult to distinguish from dementia or even delirium (see Chapter 5). When the patient happens to be delirious or demented, too, it may be impossible to determine to what degree depression is contributing to the clinical picture. Some factors (Table 7) may differentiate between depression and organic brain disease, but sometimes only a trial of treatment for depression will clarify the diagnosis.

TABLE 6. **Medications That May Cause Mania**

Baclofen

Bromocriptine

Captropril

Corticosteroids

L-dopa

Dextromethorphan

Stimulants

TABLE 7. **Depression and Dementia**

Dementia	Depression
Patient minimizes intellectual deficits	Patient advertises cognitive dysfunction
The same functions are equally impaired on different tests of the same function	Complaints of memory loss are greater than the actual deficit (e.g., the patient performs well on some tests of short-term memory but not on others)
Affect labile and shallow	Affective disturbance is pervasive
Vegetative symptoms not marked unless they are symptoms of the physical illness	Classic vegetative symptoms may be present
Past history and family history of mood disorder are less likely	Past history and family history of depression and related disorders more likely
EEG may be slower during episodes of behavioral deterioration	EEG normal
Sleep EEG normal unless the dementing illness affects the sleep–wake cycle	Sleep EEG may show decreased REM latency
Antidepressants cause increased confusion and memory loss	Antidepressants produce improvement

Somatoform disorders: In people who cannot express emotions directly, depression is often manifested by unexplained physical symptoms mixed with such subsyndromal personality characteristics as dependent clinging, manipulativeness, hostility, noncompliance, negativism, and covert resistance to attempts to help them. Because depressed mood is much less evident than its behavioral derivatives, these patients frequently appear to be suffering from primary somatization syndromes such as hypochondriasis or Briquet's syndrome (see Chapter 4). Intercurrent depression in patients who actually suffer from these disorders may be very difficult to detect because it is manifested as an increase in psychogenic somatic complaints and frustrating be-

TABLE 8. **Depression and Somatoform Disorders**

Somatoform Disorders	Depression
Vegetative symptoms less obvious	Vegetative symptoms more prominent
Physical symptoms worse at end of day	Physical symptoms may be worse in morning
Past history and family history negative for depression	Past and family history of depression and related disorders
Ill or incapacitated parent while growing up	Early loss
Symptoms appear in context of minor illness	Symptoms appear following a loss
Patient seeks out significant others and pursues multiple contacts with physicians	Patient withdraws from physicians and significant others
Patient advertises distress	Minimization or hiding of complaints
Resistance to suggestions that symptoms are psychogenic	Patient more willing to consider psychogenic etiology
Initial placebo response to antidepressants followed by return of symptoms	Positive response to antidepressants

havior. If the differential clues listed in Table 8 are not definitive, a trial of treatment for depression may be necessary to distinguish between somatization as a depressive symptom and somatization as a separate entity requiring a different therapeutic approach.

Grief: Grief (Table 9) is a normal process by which emotional investment is withdrawn from a person or thing that has been lost so that a new attachment can be formed. Initially there is a period of denial of the impact of the loss or even of the loss itself lasting from a few minutes to a few days. Many painful emotions are experienced during active grieving, which peaks in four to six weeks, is intense for three to six months, and gradually subsides over the next six months to a year. Symptoms of acute grief include waves of sadness and crying, painful preoccupation with the lost person, anxiety, an urge to search for the lost person,

TABLE 9. **Depression and Grief**

Grief	Depression
Sadness resolves when the patient expresses feelings about the loss	Only 50% of cases resolve with nonspecific encouragement to express feelings
Acute phase abates in 4–6 weeks	Spontaneous improvement takes 6–12 months
Guilt limited to feelings about what patient should have done differently or about having survived when another person has not	Pervasive guilt and self-blame
Intact self-esteem except for anxiety about living without the lost person or thing	Lowered self-esteem and self-confidence
Ends with feeling of acceptance	No sense of resolution
Recurrences primarily at important holidays and anniversaries	Recurrences become more severe and long-lasting with time
Symptoms worse in afternoon, as patient faces the day without the lost person	Symptoms worse in morning if diurnal mood variation is present

physical complaints (especially those that mimic a symptom or characteristic of the lost person), insomnia, loss of appetite, guilt about ways the patient should have behaved differently, and hallucinations of the lost person.

If the grieving patient is encouraged to express these feelings and to talk about the loss, the mourning process runs its course and normal functioning returns. A benzodiazepine sleeping pill may be prescribed, but daytime sedation blocks grieving and antidepressants make the patient feel that he or she should stop feeling sad. The patient should be reminded that sadness normally returns at significant times such as holidays and anniversaries and that no one gets over a major loss completely—nor would anyone want to do so.

Schizophrenia: Schizophrenics frequently exhibit blunted emotional expression (affect) and social withdrawal that can be confused with depression. Schizophrenic patients also become depressed, which may be masked by psychotic symptoms or mimicked by bradykinesia caused by antipsychotic drugs. On the other hand, psychotically depressed patients with bizarre and atypical psychoses may look schizophrenic. The distinction (Table 10) is important because antidepressants may aggravate schizophrenia, and antipsychotic drugs alone do not improve depression.

■ TREATMENT

Depression has an excellent prognosis when a systematic therapeutic plan is followed that involves management of suicide risk and treatment with medications and psychotherapy.

SUICIDE

Averting suicide is the first priority when treating depression (6, 18). The primary care physician is in a unique position to achieve this goal because the majority of people who kill them-

TABLE 10. **Depression and Schizophrenia**

Schizophrenia	Depression
Social withdrawal is associated with feelings of emptiness and with blunted affect	Withdrawal is associated with sadness and anxiety
No vegetative symptoms	Vegetative symptoms more common
Delusions and hallucinations not consistent with a depressed or elated mood	Delusions and hallucinations consistent with mood (e.g., delusions of guilt or sin or hallucinations telling patient to commit suicide)
Abnormal form as well as content of thinking; idiosyncratic, bizarre logic	Content of thinking is based on depressive assumptions but the form of thinking is logical
Family history of schizophrenia	Family history of depression and related disorders

selves visit their primary physicians shortly before their deaths. These patients usually do not spontaneously volunteer that they are contemplating suicide, but most disclose their intent if they are asked about suicide directly. Almost all can be cured of their suicidal thinking if a few straightforward steps are taken:

1. Ask all depressed patients about suicide. The topic can be introduced with a general question such as "are things ever so bad that life doesn't seem worth living?" If the patient replies that they have, proceed to more specific questions such as "have you thought about taking your life?"

2. Assess the immediacy of the risk. If the patient has thought of suicide, determine whether there is a concrete, feasible plan. Next, find out whether the patient has rehearsed the plan and whether there is any reason not to carry it out.

3. Assess demographic risk factors. No single factor predicts risk particularly well, but patients with a number of the risk factors listed on pp. 10–11 are in greater danger.

4. Pay attention to intuition. "Gut feelings" that the patient is suicidal frequently come from subtle nonverbal communications from the patient that the intent is greater than is apparent on the surface.

5. Hospitalize any high risk patient immediately. People may think about suicide for years, but the impulse to act usually is brief. If the patient can be prevented even temporarily from enacting a suicide plan, the urgent wish to die abates within a few hours to a week or two at most, and it disappears completely when depression is resolved. It is essential to protect the patient while treatment is being implemented.

6. Arrange involuntary hospitalization if the patient refuses to be admitted voluntarily. In most states, patients can be hospitalized against their wills if their lives are endangered by an illness such as depression that impairs their ability to appreciate that their situation is not as hopeless as they believe. The harm of hospitalizing a patient who seems to be at high risk but is later judged not to have been suicidal is much less than the harm of allowing a patient who subsequently commits suicide to refuse treatment.

7. Keep the patient under close observation until the risk abates. It does not take much ingenuity to commit suicide in a hospital, especially on a nonpsychiatric floor. The patient must be watched closely so that any actual attempts can be prevented.

8. Confront hopelessness. The extreme negative thinking of suicidal patients leads to a kind of "tunnel vision" that blinds them to obvious solutions to their problems and focuses their attention increasingly on death as the only option. It is essential that the physician not "catch" the patient's pessimism but continue to remind the patient that hopelessness is a reversible state of mind produced by a reversible disorder.

9. Maintain a close relationship with the patient. Suicidal thinking almost always remits when depression improves. The relationship with the physician provides an essential human contact and source of hope that keeps the patient alive until depression can be treated adequately.

10. Mobilize social resources. Patients frequently become suicidal because they do not know any other way to let an important person know how they feel. Unless a patient habitually uses suicidal threats as a means of influencing others, resolving a crisis in a relationship that has led to suicidal thinking usually resolves ideas of suicide. In many instances, the patient does not become suicidal again when there are further problems in the relationship.

11. Treat substance abuse, organic brain disease, and psychosis. These conditions weaken impulse control and increase the risk that the patient will not be able to refrain from acting on suicidal ideas.

DRUG THERAPY OF DEPRESSION

Antidepressants play an essential role in the treatment of depression. These drugs are most effective in reducing vegetative symptoms and psychological distress and in "unfreezing" patients who are unable to make progress in dealing with personality problems or chronic somatic complaints.

INDICATIONS

Antidepressants are used to treat depression, panic anxiety, posttraumatic stress disorder, obsessive compulsive disorder, bulimia, chronic pain, and migraine headaches (19). While there are no absolute rules, clinical experience suggests that antidepressants should be considered for depressed patients who:

- have responded to antidepressants in the past
- have vegetative symptoms
- are severely depressed
- have a family history of depression or of response of some other diagnosis to an antidepressant
- report cycles of mood, symptoms or functioning that recur in association with time of day, month, or year
- do not respond as expected to psychological interventions

MECHANISMS OF ACTION

The immediate effect of antidepressants is to increase synaptic concentrations of a number of neurotransmitters, especially norepinephrine and serotonin. Their longer-term action is to down-regulate (i.e., decrease the number of) receptors, at least to norepinephrine. In view of the many complex interactions among neuronal systems, it seems more likely that antidepressants modulate erratic functioning of multiple neurotransmitter systems than that they increase or decrease activity of any particular transmitter (15). Antidepressants also inhibit calmodulin, the intracellular protein that mediates the action of calcium ions, and some antidepressants block calcium channels (16). Whether any of the known biochemical actions of antidepressants is related to their clinical effects remains to be proven.

PREPARATIONS, DOSAGE, SIDE EFFECTS, AND INTERACTIONS

Three classes of medication are used to treat depression: cyclic antidepressants, monoamine oxidase inhibitors, and stimulants. Several other drugs are sometimes added to antidepressants to increase their effectiveness.

Cyclic Antidepressants

The heterocyclic antidepressants (Table 11) are first-line treatments for depression. All cyclic antidepressants are equally effective. Their side-effect profiles (20, 21), however, permit considerable flexibility in prescribing (Table 12). The long half-life of most cyclics (from 10–20 hours for imipramine to 80 hours for protriptyline) makes once-daily dosing possible for all prepara-

TABLE 11. **Current Available Heterocyclic Antidepressants**

Drug	Trade Name	Structure	Usual Daily Dose (mg)	Upper Daily Limit (mg)	Usual Daily Dose in Elderly (mg)
Amitriptyline[a]	Elavil	Tertiary amine	150–300	300	50–100
Nortriptyline[a]	Pamelor Aventyl	Secondary amine	75–125[b]	150[b]	25–50
Protriptyline[a]	Vivactil	Secondary amine	30–40	60	15–20
Imipramine[a]	Tofranil	Tertiary amine	150–200	300	25–100
Desipramine[a]	Norpramin Pertofane	Secondary amine	150–250	300	25–100
Trimipramine[a]	Surmontil	Tertiary amine	150–200	300	50–100
Doxepin[a]	Sinequan	Tertiary amine	150–250	300	25–50
Amoxapine[c]	Asendin	Dibenzoxazepine	150–300	600	75–300
Maprotiline[c]	Ludiomil	Tetracyclic	150–200	300	50–75
Trazodone[c]	Desyrel	Triazolopyridine	150–400	600	50–150
Bupropion[d],*	Wellbutrin	Phenylaminoketone	150–400	Not yet determined	Not yet determined
Fluoxetine[d]	Prozac	Propylamine	20–60	80	Probably 10–40

[a] Tricyclic
[b] Dosage should be adjusted according to blood level
[c] Second generation drug
[d] Third generation drug
* Not released as of March 1988

TABLE 12. **Side Effects of Heterocyclics**

Side Effects	Manifestations	Drugs
Anticholinergic	Delirium with tachycardia, warm dry skin, mydriasis	Amitriptyline, trimipramine, protriptyline, doxepin (especially when combined with other anticholinergic drugs)
Postural Hypotension (α=adrenergic)	Dizziness, unsteadiness, lightheadedness, stumbling on standing up	Tertiary amines, protriptyline, trazodone, maprotiline
Cardiovascular	Sinus tachycardia	Especially anticholinergic compounds
	Suppression of ventricular arrhythmias	
	Worsening of conduction defects	All but trazodone
	Cardiac depression (usually not significant)	
	Sinus bradycardia	Trazodone
	Worsening of ventricular arrhythmias	
Sedation	Oversedation, impaired cognition, worsening of organic brain syndrome	Amitriptyline, trimipramine, trazodone, doxepin, maprotiline
Decreased seizure threshold	Spontaneous seizures or exacerbation of epilepsy	Amoxapine, maprotiline, tertiary amines
Priapism	Priapism and rarely permanent impotence	Trazodone
Anxiety	Nervousness, tremor, sweating	Noradrenergic antidepressants (e.g., desipramine, nortriptyline), fluoxetine

Neuromuscular	Fine tremor, myoclonic jerks	Most tricyclics, maprotiline, trazodone
	Peripheral neuropathy	Amitriptyline
	Proximal myopathy	Imipramine
	Phospholipid accumulation in nerve tissue	Imipramine
Extrapyramidal	Parkinsonism, tardive dyskinesia, akathisia	Amoxapine; imipramine and amitriptyline in high doses; possibly others
Sleep changes	Increased REM latency, decreased total REM, increased stage 4, nightmares occasionally when entire dose taken at night	Most heterocyclics (except trimipramine)
Insomnia	Difficulty falling asleep	Fluoxetine, noradrenergic antidepressants
EEG changes	Suppressed alpha rhythm	Amitriptyline
	Increased synchronization at low doses	Especially tertiary amines
Hypersensitivity	Photosensitivity, eosinophilia, skin rashes	Tricyclics and maprotiline
Weight loss	Anorexia may occur, and patients with anorexia nervosa may abuse the drug to lose weight	Fluoxetine
Abstinence	Anxiety, agitation, insomnia, influenza-like symptoms	Possible with all heterocyclics on abrupt discontinuation

tions except trazodone and bupropion (22). Even though it has a half-life of 2–3 days, fluoxetine in doses greater than 20 mg/day is usually administered in divided dose and is not given at bedtime.

There can be wide interindividual variation in blood levels produced by the same dose of a given antidepressant. Clinical response correlates with blood levels (measured 10–14 hours after the last dose) only for nortriptyline, imipramine, and desipramine (23). Nortriptyline has a therapeutic window of 50–150 ng/ml (i.e., the medication does not work as well at levels above and below the window). Desipramine is more predictably effective at concentrations greater than 125 ng/ml. This drug also may have a therapeutic window, the upper level of which is not clear but probably lies somewhere between 150–200 ng/ml. The probable therapeutic concentration of imipramine plus its monodemethylated metabolite, desipramine, is 200–250 ng/ml; higher levels cause more side effects without further clinical benefit. Blood levels of all other antidepressants are used mainly to see if the serum concentration is unusually high or low, not to adjust the dose.

Patients who begin sleeping better within a week of starting an antidepressant are more likely to respond in other respects later. However, it usually takes four to six weeks for an overall clinical response to become evident. Some patients find that it may be several months before they feel completely well, and patients who have been chronically depressed may continue to note improvement over an even longer period of time. It is the clinician's task to encourage compliance during the initial phase when no response is evident yet.

Once a patient with a single depressive episode has responded, antidepressants usually are continued for 4–12 months (24). An attempt is then made to discontinue the medication slowly (e.g., by 25 mg/month of imipramine) while monitoring for return of depression. If depression returns when the dose of antidepressant is reduced, the previously effective dose should be reinstituted. Patients who have had recurrent depression or one extremely severe episode of unipolar depression should be withdrawn from antidepressants only if there is a compelling reason to do so. Abrupt withdrawal of heterocyclics can cause anorexia, nausea, vomiting, abdominal pain, diarrhea, influenza-like symptoms, insomnia, nightmares, mania, panic attacks, akathisia, and delirium (25).

Antidepressants have additive anticholinergic effects with antihistamines, antiparkinsonian drugs, and neuroleptics. Levels of cyclic antidepressants are decreased by alcohol, phenytoin, barbiturates, oral contraceptives, cigarette smoking, and chloral hydrate and increased by aspirin, phenothiazines, phenylbutazone, aminopyrine, stimulants, and scopolamine. Benzodiazepines do not alter metabolism of heterocyclics.

Monoamine oxidase inhibitors (MAOIs)

MAOIs are used to treat depression in patients who do not respond to or cannot tolerate heterocyclics. These drugs may be more effective than cyclic antidepressants in treating "atypical depression," which is accompanied by anxiety, sensitivity to rejection, self-pity, carbohydrate craving, weight gain, increased sleep, fatigue, and personality problems. MAOIs also are treatments for panic anxiety, phobic anxiety states, agoraphobia, obsessive compulsive disorder, and posttraumatic stress disorder (26, 27).

Four MAOIs are now available in the United States (Table 13). These drugs usually are administered in divided doses. With the exception of pargyline, the last dose should not be taken too

TABLE 13. **Monoamine Oxidase Inhibitors**

Generic Name	Trade Name	Class	Usual Dose (mg)	Comments
Phenelzine	Nardil	Hydrazide	45–90	Most commonly used
Isocarboxazid	Marplan	Hydrazide	20–60	More sedating
Tranylcypromine	Parnate	Non-hydrazide	20–80	Less sedation and postural hypotension; appetite suppressant; may cause hypertensive reactions without tyramine
Pargyline	Eutonyl	Non-hydrazide	25–200	Marketed as antihypertensive

late in the day or insomnia may result. About one-half of Caucasians metabolize MAOIs slowly, making them more sensitive to the drugs because of higher levels with the same dose. Rapid metabolizers, on the other hand, may need higher doses to achieve a therapeutic effect.

Of the significant side effects of MAOIs (Table 14), the most troublesome is postural hypotension. About 40% of women and an unknown number of men taking monoamine oxidase inhibitors develop anorgasmia, which occasionally is improved by cyproheptadine or urecholine. All MAOIs can cause weight gain, although tranylcypromine is least likely to be associated with this problem. Liver damage occasionally occurs with phenelzine and isocarboxazid.

It is the potential of MAOIs for dangerous interactions (28) that makes it mandatory that they only be prescribed by physicians who are familiar with their use. L-dopa, sympathetic amines, and tyramine-containing foods such as aged or processed cheese, broad bean pods, smoked and pickled foods, ripe banana skins, soy products, avocados, yeast extract, red wine and fermented beer can precipitate severe elevations in blood pressure

TABLE 14. **Adverse Effects of MAOIs**

System	Manifestations
Autonomic nervous system	Orthostatic hypotension, dry mouth, constipation, delay in micturation
Central nervous system	Toxic psychosis, insomnia, irritability, headache, ataxia
Neuromuscular	Muscle twitching, myoclonus, motor tension, tremor, muscle and joint pain, peripheral neuropathy, carpal tunnel syndrome, hyperreflexia
Liver	Jaundice, hepatocellular damage, elevated liver enzymes
Genitourinary	Impotence, anorgasmia
Miscellaneous	Edema, skin rash, blood dyscrasia (rare), aggravation of asthma, fever, constipation

(hypertensive crises) in patients taking MAOIs. Headache, fever, agitation, vomiting, chest pain, intracerebral bleeding, and heart failure may occur. Hypertensive crises are treated with oral chlorpromazine or verapamil or sublingual nifedipine before the patient reaches the hospital. The definitive treatment of sustained hypertension is 2–5 mg of intravenous phentolamine. Fatalities have been reported when MAOIs were combined with imipramine and clomipramine, and when hydrazide MAOIs were combined with nonhydrazides (28); no treatment is known for these interactions.

Stimulants

Stimulants such as methylphenidate, dextroamphetamine, and pemoline sometimes are used to treat depression in elderly, demented, and medically ill patients who cannot tolerate the standard antidepressants, and to augment the action of cyclic antidepressants in a variety of settings. A few patients develop anxiety or insomnia, but most tolerate stimulants well. Anorexia rarely occurs, and most patients with decreased appetite due to depression are able to eat and gain weight when they take a stimulant (29).

Patients who respond to stimulants usually do so in a few days. There is some debate about whether tolerance to the antidepressant effect develops, but many patients who become depressed in the context of an acute stress such as an illness can discontinue the medication when the illness begins to resolve. Dependence has not been reported in this context.

Electroconvulsive therapy (ECT)

ECT is the most effective treatment for depression. It is indicated for depression that is resistant to other therapies, severe, psychotic, or life-threatening depression, and depression in patients who cannot tolerate antidepressants. ECT also is effective for mania. ECT cures 70–80% of depressives who do not respond to antidepressants, but it does not prevent relapse. An antidepressant therefore must be administered after a successful course of ECT.

Approximately 50% of patients receiving ECT develop a transient acute organic mental syndrome, but this virtually always clears within a few hours to at most a few months. Less short-term memory loss accompanies treatment with unilateral electrodes. There is no evidence that ECT used with appropriate anesthesia causes brain damage or demonstrable permanent memory loss. *The only absolute contraindications are space-occupying lesion with increased intracranial pressure and recent carbon monoxide poisoning.* ECT has been shown to be safe in the presence of many other medical and neurological conditions and has even improved neurological status in patients with Parkinson's disease, epilepsy, and delirium (30).

Lithium

Lithium is the drug of choice for prophylaxis of recurrent mania, treatment of acute mania, and prevention of antidepressant-induced mania in depressed patients with bipolar disorder. It is controversial whether lithium can treat or prevent acute or recurrent unipolar depression, but it does appear to augment the effect of antidepressants in some depressed patients (31).

Lithium usually is given in divided dose to avoid peaks in concentration that may fall in the toxic range. The dose of lithium is always adjusted by blood level, which is measured 10–12 hours after the last dose, 5–6 days after a dosage adjustment. Acutely manic patients usually require 0.8–1.5 mEq/l, which generally is achieved at a dose of 1200–2400 mg/day. A serum concentration greater than 1.5 mEq/l almost always results in limiting side effects (32). Maintenance concentrations and levels required for an antidepressant effect appear to be in the range of 0.5–1.0 mEq/l (900–1500 mg/day), but lower doses may be effective. The dose of lithium necessary to achieve a given blood level often drops precipitously as mania is being brought under control, probably because an abnormality in a membrane lithium pump during mania that leads to intracellular accumulation of the ion is corrected as treatment progresses.

Following successful treatment of an acute episode of mania, the dose of lithium is reduced to the maintenance level and the drug is continued for a year. An attempt is then made to decrease the dose gradually, but if manic symptoms return, lithium is reinstituted. Continuous lithium therapy is necessary for patients with recurrences that are frequent or are occasional but very severe.

Common side effects of lithium (32, 33) include a fine resting tremor, myoclonus, difficulty concentrating, polyuria, poly-dipsia, goiter, hypothyroidism, nausea, diarrhea, hair loss, and hyperparathyroidism. Toxicity from excessive blood levels causes a coarse tremor, ataxia, vertigo, dysarthria, disorientation, nausea, vomiting, and coma. Sodium depletion raises serum lithium levels and hypokalemia increases the risk of side effects even at therapeutic lithium concentrations. Hypothyroidism, which may be induced by lithium treatment, can aggravate lithium toxicity.

Lithium levels are raised by sodium-wasting diuretics and tetracycline and lowered by potassium-sparing diuretics. Lithium and calcium channel blocking agents have additive effects on the cardiac conduction system. A good deal of concern has been expressed about potential interactions with neuroleptics and carbamazepine. This issue is addressed in Chapter 7.

A number of experimental alternatives to lithium have been introduced for patients who cannot tolerate or do not respond to lithium. The best studied of these have been ECT, carbamazepine, verapamil, reserpine, clonazepam, and lorazepam (33, 34).

SELECTION OF AN ANTIDEPRESSANT

There are a few simple guidelines for the prescription of antidepressant medications:

1. Use a drug to which the patient has responded in the past. The same medication is often effective again; however, some patients who had a good response to a particular drug during one or more previous episodes do not benefit from it during a subsequent episode and need another drug instead.

2. Prescribe a medication to which a family member has responded. Inherited patterns of metabolism predict that a response is more likely if the patient has a blood relative who has improved with the same drug.

3. Select a secondary amine, trazodone, stimulant, or ECT for patients who cannot tolerate sedation, postural hypotension, or anticholinergic side effects. Elderly and demented patients and patients with glaucoma and prostatism do better with these treatments.

4. Give trazodone to patients who are sensitive to the quinidine-like effect of the other cyclic antidepressants. However, trazodone can aggravate ventricular irritability while the other cyclics reduce it. Trazodone also has caused priapism leading to irreversible impotence in a small number of patients.

5. *Minimize the use of tranquilizers for depressed patients who are also anxious.* Antianxiety drugs may improve compliance with antidepressants during the first month of therapy, but in the long run they aggravate depression. Sedating antidepressants (e.g., amitryptiline, trazodone, doxepin) and MAOIs are often more useful than antianxiety drug–antidepressant combinations. Antidepressants that increase brain norepinephrine levels, such as desipramine and nortriptyline, may lead to increased anxiety early in treatment.

6. *Consider stimulants for demented or physically ill patients.* ECT also is safe in dementia and may even improve delirium (30).

7. *Do not give maprotiline or amoxapine to epileptic patients.* These drugs lower the seizure threshold substantially. Secondary amines, doxepin, and MAOIs are safer for patients with seizure disorders. Bupropion and fluoxetine may cause spontaneous seizures.

8. *Add neuroleptics to antidepressants when treating psychotic depression.* Depression accompanied by delusions, hallucinations, or severe disorganization is much more likely to respond to drug combinations or to ECT than to antidepressants or neuroleptics alone. Amoxapine, which has neuroleptic properties, is effective by itself.

9. *Consider MAOIs for depression accompanied by personality disorder, severe anxiety, hypersomnia, increased appetite and weight, and reverse diurnal mood swing.* Cyclic antidepressants may be effective in atypical depression, but MAOIs may be more beneficial.

WHAT IF THE PATIENT DOES NOT RESPOND?

Approximately 70% of depressed patients respond to cyclic antidepressants. Other antidepressants, drug combinations, and ECT increase the rate of improvement to 80–85% of those who do not commit suicide, but 15% do not recover. Treatment resistant patients can be approached with the following questions:

1. Is the patient really depressed? The patient may really have a personality disorder or other psychiatric condition that is mistaken for depression.

2. Is a medical illness, medication, nonprescription drug, or alcohol interfering with the response to therapy? Alcohol, tranquilizers, drugs that lower antidepressant blood levels (e.g., oral contraceptives), anemia, and subclinical hypothyroidism are common culprits. An illness may be mild from a medical standpoint and still be responsible for failure to respond to an antidepressant.

3. Have I prescribed an adequate dose of antidepressant? The most common cause of treatment failure is inadequate dosage. If an unresponsive patient is not experiencing significant side effects, increasing the dose toward the maximum recommended level (Table 12) may result in improvement. Patients taking nortriptyline and possibly desipramine require a reduction in dose if the blood level is above the therapeutic window.

4. Has the patient had an adequate trial of medication? It can take six weeks or more at a therapeutic dose before the patient responds; it is a mistake to change the drug before that point if the patient is tolerating an adequate dose. On the other hand, there is no point in continuing an antidepressant that clearly has been of no benefit after a good therapeutic trial. In this case, the medication should be changed from one class of tricyclic to another (e.g., from nortriptyline to desipramine) or from a first generation to a newer generation drug (e.g., from amitryptiline to maprotiline). Patients who do not respond to cyclic antidepressants may do better with MAOIs, as may those with atypical depression.

5. Is the patient taking the medication? Hopelessness, guilt, fear of what things would be like if the patient were not depressed, and intolerance of side effects make many depressed patients noncompliant. It is therefore important to question patients repeatedly about compliance. Blood levels that are exceptionally low for a given dose suggest either rapid metabolism or noncompliance.

6. Should the antidepressant be augmented? Four agents can be added to antidepressants to increase their effectiveness. Each is useful about one-third of the time:

- Lithium in a dose of 600–1200 μg/day usually leads to a response within a week or two, although it may take up to a month
- Stimulants (e.g., methylphenidate 10–40 mg/day) usually augment the antidepressant within a few days to a week. Older patients may be more responsive
- T_3 in a dose of 25–50 μg has been used by some clinicians to increase the effectiveness of antidepressants. It is not clear whether this approach is more effective in patients who are subclinically hypothyroid
- Tryptophan or 5-hydroxytryptophan occasionally augment the action of an antidepressant, possibly by increasing brain levels of serotonin. The usual dose is 1–3 grams, but some clinicians use higher doses. Pyrodixine is a necessary cofactor. The "serotonin syndrome," which consists of confusion, psychosis, and cerebellar signs may occur when higher doses of tryptophan are combined with antidepressants, especially with MAOIs.

7. Is the patient psychotic? Patients with psychotic depression require ECT or a combination of a neuroleptic and an antidepressant.

8. Is the medication making the patient worse? Antidepressants speed up the inherent tendency of depression to remit. In some patients, especially those with bipolar disorder, they also can increase the tendency of depression to recur (35). In patients who have recurrent cycles of mania and depression or who experience increasingly frequent episodes of depression, the antidepressant may cure each episode only to make the patient cycle quickly into another episode. Adding carbamazepine or thyroid hormone, or discontinuing the antidepressant, may slow this cycling. If it does not, or if depression becomes more severe, ECT may be necessary.

9. Does the patient need ECT? Patients become responsive to previously ineffective medications after ECT.

10. Does someone else want the patient to remain depressed? "Significant others" who are accustomed to the patient's depression, have their own theories about its cause, or feel left out of the treatment may encourage depressive behaviors in the patient. These factors can only be evaluated by including those important to the patient in therapy whenever feasible.

11. Am I paying more attention to the patient's body than the patient's mind? People who feel that the physician is only interested in signs, symptoms, and medications may express their need to talk more about themselves in the form of continued depression and side effects that force the physician to adjust medications and otherwise interact with them.

■ NEW NONPHARMACOLOGIC PHYSICAL TREATMENTS FOR DEPRESSION

In recent years, several innovative biological treatments for depression have been introduced that do not involve medications or ECT. These treatments are not more effective than the standard ones; but they are more acceptable to people who do not like medications or who have intolerable side effects. Pregnant women also may prefer one of these therapies.

BRIGHT LIGHT THERAPY

Artificial light of the approximate intensity of sunlight (2500 lux) ameliorates seasonal affective disorder within a few days; discontinuation of light therapy for more than two or three days results in relapse. When it is started early in the fall, light therapy also prevents winter depression. Commercial units are available, or the patient may wish to construct a cheaper model from six four-foot florescent lights or "Vita Lights." Two hours of exposure sitting within a meter of the light and glancing at it about once per minute seems to be the minimum effective initial dosage, although it may be possible to reduce the amount of light exposure after the patient has responded. It is not clear whether the timing of the light (e.g., in the morning for patients who sleep late and in the afternoon for those who wake up early) is crucial to a clinical response, so most clinicians advise the patient to experiment and find the time or times that seem to work best (35).

SLEEP DEPRIVATION

One night's sleep deprivation may dramatically improve 50% of depressed patients. Unfortunately, the patient feels even worse after recovery sleep the following night. A more practical approach is depriving the patient of sleep during the second half of the night only (when most REM sleep occurs) or attempting to reduce REM sleep only.

SLEEP PHASE CHANGES

Some experts advocate attempting to correct phase shifts in biological rhythms in depression by changing sleep times (35). For example, if the patient usually wakes up early in the morning, the patient is assumed to have a phase advance of the sleep cycle that results in the brain falling asleep and waking up early with respect to the actual time of day. Manipulating sleep in the opposite direction—in this example by having the patient stay up later and sleep later the next morning—may reset the sleep cycle and in some instances may improve depression.

■ WHAT TO SAY TO DEPRESSED PATIENTS

Some people think that talking to depressed patients is complicated and time-consuming. The fact is that brief and focused approaches that are easily adapted to the office or hospital can be highly effective. Any clinician treating depression should be familiar with at least some of the techniques that have been shown to benefit depressed patients (17, 18, 36, 37).

Establish a Positive, Supportive Relationship. Even if depression is not caused by a problem in a relationship, it causes problems in relationships. The emotional connection to the clinician is crucial in providing a forum for resolving feelings about other important interactions and in maintaining the patient's hope and confidence.

See the Patient Regularly. Depressed people are highly sensitive to loss and rejection. "As needed" appointments or hospital visits whose length is proportional to how badly the patient feels make the patient uncertain about the stability of the doctor–patient relationship while demonstrating that it is possible to hold onto the doctor through suffering. The duration of appointments (15–30 minutes is sufficient in nonpsychiatric practice) should be understood by the patient in advance in order to minimize feeling rejected when meetings end.

Be Hopeful. Patients feel misunderstood and emotionally

abandoned by glib, superficial reassurances. However, it is crucial to avoid being contaminated by the depressed patient's unrealistic pessimism. At least some of this negativism is a test of whether the physician really believes that the patient can get better. Remind the patient that even though the patient may not believe it, the physician has a treatment that has a high rate of cure if patient and physician persist with it.

Set Realistic Goals. People become depressed when they fail to live up to unrealistic expectations of themselves. To prevent the patient from doing the same thing in treatment, concrete, finite goals should be agreed upon. Looking in the want ads is a more immediate first step, for example, than finding a job. Patients who believe that they must either be totally well or completely ill should be reminded of the improvement they have made when they interpret a minor setback as a sign that they have made no progress at all.

Confront Negative Thinking. One way of overcoming the depressive tendency to draw globally negative conclusions from experiences that are not as bad as the patient thinks is to have the patient keep a record of situations in which depression is experienced. The patient is then asked to write down what he or she was thinking when feeling depressed and to generate alternative thoughts that are inconsistent with depression. For example, if a man's wife seems to ignore him when he comes home from work, he might conclude that she was angry with him. Next, he might decide that she was always angry, and that she was angry because she did not love him. Such a patient would be asked to write down alternative explanations for his observations; for example, that his wife was not angry but distracted, that she was angry at someone else, that she was only angry about a specific incident, or that she could only be angry at him if she cared enough about him to be upset by him. The next step would be to explore the underlying belief that led to the patient's negative idea; for example, that if people are not unequivocally positive about him, they are unequivocally negative.

Facilitate Grieving. Unresolved grief should be dealt with by confronting reluctance to deal with the pain of grief and then by encouraging the patient to express feelings about the loss.

Encourage the Expression of Anger. Patients turn anger inward because they feel guilty or because they are afraid that their anger will hurt or drive away the people they need. These patients can practice with the physician how to talk about anger without feeling overwhelmed and then can tell the people who are actually involved about how they feel. It may be helpful to have the physician present when the patient first begins to express anger openly to others.

Involve the Family. A spouse or other important individual should always be included in treatment if the patient's complaint includes not being able to get along with that person. Even when patients have no stated concerns about other people, it is a good idea at least to evaluate family members' interactions with them and review the family's view of how the patient is doing, which may differ drastically from the patient's view. Important goals for the family may include:

- *Treating depression in significant others.* Assortative mating and genetic influences make depression in the family and loved ones of depressed patients a common problem that needs to be addressed.
- *Exploring anger.* The family may be angry with the patient's passivity, provocations, or failure to improve. If they are afraid that expressing their anger openly will make the patient feel more depressed, they may express it covertly through withdrawal or negative statements about the treatment.
- *Confronting manipulation.* Patients who become depressed when they should feel angry or assertive may be using unhappiness as a way of influencing people whom they feel helpless to deal with in more direct ways. If the family is helped to confront this behavior without fear that the patient will respond by getting worse, the patient will be forced to find more constructive approaches to meeting important needs.
- *Negotiating role disputes.* A common modern marital misunderstanding is the expectation that a woman who is at home with the children should do all the housework even though she hates it, while the husband's role does not necessarily involve interacting with the children or talking about his feelings. Frequently, such role expectations are assumed by both parties without their ever having discussed the issue openly. Attempting to satisfy someone else's unrealistic expectation leads to

depression, whereas openly discussing feelings about important roles results in new roles that feel better to both parties.

Re-evaluate Suicide Risk. A patient may be too depressed to commit suicide at one point only to become a serious risk when increasing energy levels make suicide feasible. Another patient may relapse when antidepressant levels change or after encountering a disappointment that stimulates the belief that since everything is no longer perfect it must be hopeless. It is therefore essential to re-evaluate suicidal thoughts and plans periodically, especially when the patient suddenly seems to feel better for no apparent reason, relapses, becomes preoccupied with people who have died or with potential means of suicide, makes out a will in the middle of treatment, plans an unexpected trip, or gives some other clue that makes the physician feel instinctively that the patient might be suicidal.

■ REFERENCES

1. Weissman MM, Merikangas KR, Boyd JH: Epidemiology of affective disorders, in Psychiatry. Edited by Michaels R, Cavenar JO, Brodie HKH, et al. Philadelphia, J.B. Lippincott, 1986
2. Wehr TA, Goodwin FK: Circadian Rhythms in Psychiatry. Pacific Grove, CA, The Boxwood Press, 1983
3. Weissman MM, Wickramaritne P, Merikangas KB, et al: Onset of major depression in early adulthood. Arch Gen Psychiatry 1984; 41:1136–1139
4. Whybrow PC, Akiskal HS, Mckinney WT: Mood Disorders: Toward a New Psychobiology. New York, Plenum Press, 1984
5. Wender PH, Kety SS, Rosenthal D: Psychiatric disorders in the biological and adoptive families of adopted individuals with affective disorders. Arch Gen Psychiatry 1986; 43:923–929
6. Murphy GE: Suicide and attempted suicide, in Psychiatry. Edited by Michels R, Cavenar JO, Brodie HKH, et al. Philadelphia, J.B. Lippincott, 1986
7. Robins E: The Final Months. New York, Oxford University Press, 1981
8. Shapiro MF, Lehman AF, Greenfield S: Biases in the laboratory diagnosis of depression in medical practice. Arch Intern Med 1983; 143:2985–3088

9. Arana GW, Barrera PJ, Cohen BM, et al: The dexasmethasone suppression test in psychotic disorders. Am J Psychiatry 1983; 140:1521–1523

10. Pitts FN: Recent research on the DST. J Clin Psychiatry 1984; 45:380–381

11. Loosen PT, Prange AJ: Serum thyrotropin response to thyrotropin releasing hormone in psychiatric patients: a review. Am J Psychiatry 1982; 139:505–516

12. Kupfer DJ, Foster FG, Coble P, et al: The application of sleep EEG for the differential diagnosis of affective disorders. Am J Psychiatry 1978; 135:69–74

13. Akiskal HS: Dysthymic disorder: Psychopathology of proposed chronic depressive subtypes. Am J Psychiatry 1983; 140:11–20

14. Ross ED, Rush AJ: Diagnosis and neuroanatomical correlates of depression in brain damaged patients. Arch Gen Psychiatry 1981; 38:1344–1354

15. Siever LJ, Davis KL: Overview: toward a dysregulation hypothesis of depression. Am J Psychiatry 1985; 142:1017–1031

16. Dubovsky SL, Franks RD: Intracellular calcium ions in affective disorders. Biol Psychiatry 1983; 18:783–797

17. Beck A, Rush AJ: Cognitive Therapy of Depression. New York, Guilford, 1979

18. Dubovsky SL, Weissberg MP: Clinical Psychiatry in Primary Care, 3rd edition. Baltimore, Williams & Wilkins, 1986

19. Goodman WK, Charney DS: Therapeutic applications and mechanisms of action of monamine oxidase and heterocyclic antidepressant drugs. J Clin Psychiatry 1985; 46:6–22

20. Richelson E: The newer antidepressants. Psychopharmacol Bull 1984; 20:213–223

21. Fiori MG: Tricyclic antidepressants: a review of their toxicity. Curr Dev Psychopharmacol 1977; 4:72–94

22. Baldessarini RJ: Drugs and the treatment of psychiatric disorders, in The Pharmacologic Basis of Therapeutics. Edited by Gilman AG, Goodman LS, Rall TW, et al. Macmillan, 1985

23. Task Force on the Use of Laboratory Tests in Psychiatry: Tricyclic antidepressants: blood level measurements and clinical outcome. Am J Psychiatry 1985; 142:155–162

24. Prien RF, Kupfer DJ: Continuation drug therapy for major depressive episodes: how long should it be maintained? Am J Psychiatry 1986; 143:18–23

25. Lawrence JM: Reactions to withdrawal of antidepressants, antiparkinsonian drugs and lithium. Psychosomatics 1985; 11:869–877

26. Pare CMB: The present status of monoamine oxidase inhibitors. Br J Psychiatry 1985; 146:576–584

27. Klein DF, Gittleman R, Quitkin F, et al: Diagnosis and Drug Treatment of Psychiatric Disorders: Adults and Children. Baltimore, Williams & Wilkins, 1980

28. Hansten PD: Drug Interactions, 5th edition. Philadelphia, Lea and Febiger, 1985

29. Kaufman MW, Cassem N, Murray G, et al: The use of methylphenidate in depressed patients after cardiac surgery. J Clin Psychiatry 1984; 45:82–84

30. Dubovsky SL: Using electroconvulsive therapy in patients with neurological disease. Hosp Community Psychiatry 1986; 37:819–825

31. Garbutt JC, Mayo JP, Gillette GM, et al: Lithium potentiation of tricyclic antidepressants following lack of T_3 potentiation in treatment resistant depression. Am J Psychiatry 1986; 143:1038–1039

32. Jefferson JW, Griest JH: Primer of lithium therapy, 2nd edition. Baltimore, Williams & Wilkins, 1986

33. Dubovsky SL, Ringel SP: Psychopharmacologic treatment in neurological practice. J Neuro Rehab 1987; 2:51–66

34. Dubovsky SL: Calcium antagonists: a new class of psychiatric drugs? Psychiatr Ann 1986; 16:724–728

35. Wehr TA, Goodwin FK: Can antidepressants worsen the course of affective illness? Am J Psychiatry 1987; 144:1403–1411

36. Karasu TB: The Psychiatric Therapies. Washington DC, American Psychiatric Press, 1984

37. Weissman MM, Klerman GL, Prusoff BA, et al: Depressed outpatients: results one year after therapy with drugs and/or interpersonal therapy. Arch Gen Psychiatry 1981; 38:51–55

ANANTY 2

Anxiety is ubiquitous in medical practice and in the population at large. As many as 35% of otherwise healthy people have had sporadic panic attacks, and 0.4–1.6% of the general population have panic attacks frequently enough to warrant a diagnosis of panic disorder. Severe phobias and agoraphobia (fear of leaving the familiarity of the home) occur in 1.2–5.8% of all people, while as many as 19% have milder phobias. Generalized anxiety afflicts 4% of Americans (1).

Like depression, anxiety is frequently misdiagnosed and inadequately treated. One group of 100 patients with panic attacks, for example, had accumulated a total of 215 years of psychotherapy and had taken over 1 million doses of tranquilizers prescribed by an average of 10 physicians per patient. Twenty years later, 90% of the patients were still incapacitated (2).

■ ANXIETY AND FEAR

Anxiety is like fear in that it involves mental and physical mobilization to meet a perceived danger. Unlike fear, anxiety does not arise in response to an identifiable threat or if it does, it is out of proportion to the actual stimulus and persists after the objective danger subsides. Moderate levels of anxiety facilitate adaptation, as when someone who worries about failing an examination studies harder. Excessive levels of anxiety, however, paralyze mental resources in a morass of continuous and futile mobilizations of mind and body.

■ SIGNS AND SYMPTOMS

Anxiety is manifested by mental, behavioral, and physical symptoms.

EMOTIONAL SYMPTOMS

Anxious people are fearful, easily panicked, irritable, and impatient; many are also depressed. When mental defenses against anxiety predominate, the patient is more aware of feeling numb, unreal, and detached as all mental experience is dampened in an attempt to dampen anxiety. The constant mental arousal of anxiety may lead to a feeling of fatigue, inner depletion, and inability to rise to a challenge.

THINKING

The thoughts of the anxious person are oriented toward uncertainty and danger. The patient is hypervigilant and preoccupied, convinced that the worst is always about to happen, fearful of losing control, and exquisitely alert to minor physical dysfunction and medication side effects that most people would ignore. Through repeated questions to which the answers are obvious, the anxious patient elicits support and reassurance, while at the same time doubting the physician's assessments and advice, for example by asking "Are you *sure* that this drug is safe?" Severe anxiety is a disorganizing experience, so many anxious patients have difficulty concentrating and impaired performance on tests of memory and intellectual functioning.

BEHAVIOR

Anxious patients become increasingly unwilling to venture away from home or from other familiar places in which they feel comfortable, to avoid settings that threaten them with novelty or psychological stimulation. They startle easily, lack self-confidence, and avoid taking chances. They may be outgoing in one-on-one situations but inhibited and shy in groups. Social anxiety may prevent them from advancing in careers that require public speaking, performing, or writing.

PHYSICAL SYMPTOMS

Physical complaints, which usually represent heightened awareness of arousal of the sympathetic nervous system and motor tension, are common in anxious patients. Typical symptoms include insomnia, nausea, diarrhea, abdominal pain, difficulty swallowing, dry mouth, hot flashes, urinary frequency, sexual dysfunction, faintness, tremor, muscle tension and soreness, fatigue, headaches, diaphoresis, cold, clammy hands, palpitations, and chest pain. Hyperventilation produced by anxiety causes shortness of breath, dizziness, lightheadedness, numbness, and paresthesias.

■ CATEGORIES OF ANXIETY

Anxiety may be limited to specific circumstances, or it may not be confined to any particular situation. Anxiety disorders in the latter group include panic disorder, generalized anxiety disorder, and obsessive compulsive disorder. Anxiety disorders that are more situation-specific include phobias, posttraumatic stress disorder, and certain types of anxiety that are aroused by medical illness.

PANIC DISORDER

Panic disorder is characterized by discrete, abrupt, unprovoked attacks of intense paroxysmal anxiety, usually accompanied by autonomic arousal. Panic attacks typically last a few minutes and abate rapidly but are so intense that they are extremely disruptive. Repeated panic attacks often evoke anticipatory anxiety, or fear of having more panic attacks. Patients with acute panic attacks may also have chronic anxiety that does not reach the threshold for a full-blown panic attack (subpanic anxiety) that is manifested as unease, edginess, feelings of detachment, and physical symptoms of low-grade arousal such as knots in the stomach, headaches, neurological complaints, and lightheadedness.

GENERALIZED ANXIETY DISORDER

Generalized anxiety disorder is the formal diagnostic term for anxiety lasting more than six months concerning two or more events (e.g., health, academic performance, loved ones) about which there is no actual cause for intense worry. At least six typical physical and/or psychological symptoms of anxiety must be continuously present to make this diagnosis in the current nomenclature.

OBSESSIVE COMPULSIVE DISORDER

This condition, which has a lifetime prevalence of 2–3%, is classified with the anxiety disorders because anxiety becomes intolerable when the patient attempts to resist obsessions or compulsions. Many depressed and anxious people have mild obsessions (recurrent, intrusive, senseless ideas that the patient recognizes as the products of his or her mind and actively but unsuccessfully attempts to resist) and compulsions (repetitive, purposeful behaviors performed in accordance with an obsession or a stereotyped rule that is designed to neutralize some terrible consequence in a magical way). When these symptoms by themselves significantly interfere with functioning or are markedly time-consuming, a separate disorder requiring specialized treatment is diagnosed.

PHOBIAS

Phobias are persistent, unrealistic fears of situations that are compulsively avoided, even though the patient knows that there is no actual reason to fear them. There are three types of phobias:

AGORAPHOBIA

This is fear of being without a familiar figure in circumstances or places from which escape might be difficult or embarrassing or in which help might not be available. Agoraphobic patients may avoid crowds, bridges, elevators, public transportation, driving, or sitting in the middle of a row of seats in a theater. In severe cases only the home feels safe, and the patient becomes housebound. Agoraphobia usually develops in patients who have repeated panic attacks that make them fearful of experiencing, in any situation that does not feel completely safe, the feeling of incapacitation that accompanies bouts of panic anxiety (3).

SOCIAL PHOBIA

Social phobia is a persistent fear of being humiliated in public. It may involve a specific inhibition (e.g., fear of public speaking) or more global fears of social interactions.

SIMPLE PHOBIAS

These are unrealistic fears of specific, circumscribed situations or things such as dogs or heights.

POSTTRAUMATIC STRESS DISORDER (PTSD)

PTSD is a persistent state of mental and physical arousal lasting for at least one month, which develops in response to an unusual stress that most people would be expected to find extremely disturbing, such as an accident, assault, or natural disaster. PTSD may begin immediately after the trauma, or its onset may be delayed six months or more. Specific symptoms include hypervigilance, irritability, exaggerated startle response, insomnia, recurrent intrusive recollections and dreams about the event, avoidance of situations that recall the trauma, intense distress upon exposure to events that symbolize or recall the trauma, and various forms of psychic and emotional numbing that are common in people who avoid anxiety by avoiding all feelings.

SITUATION-SPECIFIC ANXIETY IN MEDICALLY ILL PATIENTS

Certain types of anxiety that arise in response to specific situations or conflicts are not formal diagnostic entities, but they may underlie common problem behaviors in some patients, especially in the medically ill.

SEPARATION ANXIETY

This is distress that is experienced when the patient is separated from an important caretaker or other supportive figure. Separation anxiety may take the form of outright fearfulness, disruptive behavior, physical complaints, and increased demands for attention, such as repeatedly asking to see a doctor or ringing for the nurse whenever the patient is left alone. Separation anxiety is normal in young children; it is also seen in adults who function at a childhood psychological level (i.e., who are regressed), as may occur during physical illness or other times of major stress.

STRANGER ANXIETY

Another normal experience in childhood, stranger anxiety, may also be experienced by regressed adults. It is manifested by distress or increased complaints when the patient is confronted by unfamiliar physicians or caretakers.

ANXIETY ABOUT DEPENDENCY

This may be masked by a facade of excessive autonomy and self-sufficiency in people who are attempting to avoid awareness of a strong underlying need to depend on others. These individuals are threatened by any situation that makes them feel dependent (e.g., an illness) and attempt to prove that they do not need anyone by devaluing those who offer help and by refusing to comply with the treatment.

ANXIETY ABOUT LOSS OF CONTROL

This type of anxiety drives some patients to attempt to control every aspect of their illness and its treatment. These patients are threatened when important decisions are taken out of their hands, for example when they require hospitalization. Arguing about the diagnosis or treatment, noncompliance and failure to keep appointments may be attempts to assert themselves in opposition to the doctor in order to regain a sense of control.

ANXIETY ABOUT THE MEANING OF AN ILLNESS

Any illness can arouse worries about loss of function, beauty, abandonment, pain, or about death. The patient may be obviously anxious, or the anxiety may be partially hidden by the patient's attempts at self-reassurance. For example, the patient who fears that others will only love him if he is well may alienate loved ones to drive them off before they decide to leave on their own; or the patient who is worried about no longer being attractive may engage in inappropriately seductive behavior.

SIGNAL ANXIETY

Signal anxiety is anxiety that signals the threatened emergence of thoughts, desires, impulses, or emotions that have been kept out of awareness because a patient has learned that they are bad or could result in adverse consequences such as hurting someone or being abandoned, disliked, or humiliated. Signal anxiety may be evoked by any event that has important symbolic meaning, making an inherently benign situation feel inappropriately frightening.

■ PRESENT ILLNESS

Forms of anxiety are differentiated from each other through careful history taking. Important areas to assess include:

1. When does the patient feel anxious? Anxiety that occurs in only one setting suggests a phobia, PTSD, or reaction to illness. Anxiety that occurs primarily in the context of an important relationship signals a conflict in the relationship. Patients who are less anxious when around familiar people may have agoraphobia, separation anxiety, or delirium.

2. Does the patient have panic attacks? Discrete, unprovoked bouts of intense anxiety and autonomic arousal require a different treatment than do other forms of anxiety. The patient may be less aware of panic attacks than of ongoing subpanic and anticipatory anxiety. Patients whose behavior has become severely restricted and patients with multiple phobias should be questioned closely about panic attacks, as should any patient who is depressed.

3. Has the patient had a traumatic experience? Relatively minor stresses in the present (e.g., a close call in an accident in which there were no injuries) may reactivate unresolved PTSD from previous traumas. The diagnosis of PTSD therefore should not be discounted just because a recent experience has not been overwhelming.

4. How does the patient feel about a medical illness? Anxiety that develops in the context of a medical or surgical illness should be evaluated by asking the patient and the family about the patient's feelings regarding the condition and its treatment.

5. Is the patient also depressed? Anxiety and depression frequently accompany each other and affect each other's manifestations, course, and response to treatment.

■ PAST HISTORY

Patients with panic anxiety may have a history of severe separation anxiety or school phobia in childhood. Panic attacks tend to begin in the late teens or twenties. Panic attacks usually become more frequent with time, and phobic avoidance develops as the patient experiences panic and anticipatory anxiety in a growing variety of situations. Panic may remit spontaneously, but it usually returns unless appropriate treatment is instituted.

■ FAMILY HISTORY

Panic disorder appears to have a genetic component; genetic influences are less clear in generalized anxiety disorder (4). The likelihood of a genetically transmitted vulnerability is greater in anxious patients with both panic attacks and depression in the family and in those with a younger age of onset of anxiety. Anxious patients with a family history of depression are more likely to become depressed as well as anxious, while those whose blood relatives suffer only from anxiety are more likely to suffer only from anxiety.

■ ASSOCIATED PROBLEMS

Any anxious patient should be evaluated for conditions that commonly accompany anxiety.

DEPRESSION

Approximately 70–80% of cases of depression are accompanied by significant anxiety, and 30% of apparent anxiety disorders mask an underlying depression. Between four- and nine-tenths of people who suffer from panic attacks become depressed, too, and 20% of depressives eventually have panic attacks. Patients with panic disorder psychologically are similar to depressed patients, even before they become symptomatic. The presence of depression affects treatment decisions in anxiety disorders, since many antianxiety drugs can aggravate depression, while antidepressants improve some forms of anxiety. However, ECT, which is very useful for depression, is of no benefit in primary anxiety states.

SUBSTANCE ABUSE

Attempts at self-treatment with alcohol and tranquilizers can lead to a vicious circle of escalating abuse. Central nervous system (CNS) depressants temporarily relieve anxiety, but withdrawal a few hours later increases anxiety, in response to which the patient increases the dose, causing more intense withdrawal later that requires an even higher dose. When people use tranquilizers, alcohol, or other drugs to feel more comfortable in social settings, they end up interacting only when they are intoxicated and do not have an opportunity to learn other ways of relating.

WITHDRAWAL AND AVOIDANCE

As they become less confident in themselves, many anxious patients begin to avoid situations in which they must perform, function socially, assert themselves, or risk danger or embarrassment. The less experience they have in these settings, the more insecure and anxious they become.

DEPENDENCY

Whenever a person is frightened it is natural to want to lean on anyone who can offer support and reassurance. Even people who have been strong-willed and independent may become reluctant to do anything by themselves. Eventually, they may insist that their spouses or children accompany them everywhere.

HYPOCHONDRIASIS

Anxious patients worry about whatever issue is most important to them. If they have somatic symptoms of hyperventilation, autonomic arousal, or a benign physical illness, they may decide that they have some serious disease that the physician has overlooked or that a condition that they actually have is much worse then the doctor thinks. Reassurance is only of transient benefit until the underlying anxiety is treated, because the patient feels that the doctor does not understand the seriousness of the situation or is concealing the terrible truth.

MARITAL AND FAMILY PROBLEMS

When spouses become impatient with the patient's avoidance, withdrawal, insecurity, and dependency, they may attempt to pressure the anxious patient into becoming more functional. When the patient attempts to comply by forcing himself into situations that evoke anxiety, the connection between those situations and feeling anxious is strengthened, making the situation worse. Children of anxious patients may be thrust into a protective parent role, to which they react with premature pseudomaturity or with anxiety, rebellion, and substance abuse.

MITRAL VALVE PROLAPSE (MVP)

MVP is found with greater frequency in patients with panic disorder than in the general population. While some symptoms of MVP (e.g., palpitations and lightheadedness) may mimic anxiety symptoms, MVP does not cause panic attacks. The principal reason for evaluating panic patients for MVP is to be alert for the rare medical complications of MVP that may occur (5).

■ LABORATORY FINDINGS

Several substances have been used to provoke anxiety in various settings. These tests are either too invasive or experimental to be appropriate for clinical diagnosis, but they illustrate the fact that anxiety depends on mechanisms of the body as well as mechanisms of the mind.

LACTATE

The intravenous infusion of sodium lactate precipitates panic attacks in roughly 70% of patients with panic disorder (2). When the panic disorder is successfully treated, lactate loses its ability to evoke panic. Several possible explanations for this phenomenon have been proposed, but the actual mechanism remains unknown.

YOHIMBINE

Yohimbine is a drug that blocks α_2 autoreceptors located on presynaptic noradrenergic neurons, many of which are located in the major alerting center of the brain, the locus coeruleus (described below). The α_2 autoreceptor is a regulatory mechanism that shuts down production and release of norepinephrine as levels in the synapse rise. Blocking the autoreceptor increases activity of this transmitter, thereby "turning up the volume" of the locus coeruleus and activating the brain. Patients with panic disorder who are given yohimbine develop panic attacks, suggesting that the panic attacks are related to excessive activity of noradrenergic circuits in the locus coeruleus (6).

BETA-CARBOLINE-3-CARBOXYLIC ACID (BETA-CCE)

Beta-CCE interferes with the action of the benzodiazepine receptor complex in the brain (described below). It produces agitation in animals and extreme generalized anxiety in the few people who have taken it (7).

BETA ADRENERGIC AGONISTS

Isoproterenol evokes or aggravates anxiety in anxiety-prone patients; other people simply feel physically uncomfortable. There may be a two-way association between physiologic arousal and anxiety, so that the tachycardia produced by beta agonists calls forth anxiety as a conditioned response. Another possibility is that stimulation of brain beta receptors may somehow be involved in the anxiety response.

■ COURSE

Anxiety that is specific to a reversible situation such as an acute illness usually abates when the situation changes. Signal anxiety may lead to a new and better adaptation if conflicts that were kept out of awareness prior to the crisis come into awareness and are resolved. Without treatment, panic anxiety tends to get worse with time. Untreated PTSD is frequently chronic or relapsing, especially if there were severe or multiple traumas or if the traumatic situation involved engaging in activities that the patient continues to consider reprehensible.

■ ETIOLOGY

Anxiety can best be conceptualized as an organismic warning of danger or a situation that is sufficiently unfamiliar that it could be dangerous. The danger may be objective or symbolic, external or internal, conscious or unconscious. The signal of danger may arise in the mind, in which case a specific psychological meaning can be uncovered, or it may be initiated by a malfunction in brain substrates for anxiety. In this case, the patient may attempt to understand what is essentially a contentless experience by explaining the anxiety on the basis of some important conflict.

PSYCHOLOGICAL FACTORS

It is the perception and meaning of a danger, and not its inherent severity, that determines whether a person becomes anxious. What seems trivial to one person may have overwhelming significance to another. Conflicts that cannot be resolved by one's usual problem-solving methods create uncertainty and therefore arouse anxiety. An anxiogenic conflict may be between different desires, or between an impulse to do or feel something and the sense that it will result in guilt, retaliation, or pain.

Anxiety can be learned when a benign situation becomes associated with something that causes anxiety. Anxiety may then generalize to any situation that resembles the original stimulus. For example, a patient who had a bad experience in one hospital may become afraid of all hospitals. The very thought of becoming ill then arouses anxiety because of the danger that it might lead to hospitalization.

BIOLOGICAL FACTORS

Interest in the biology of anxiety has focused on the locus coeruleus, a small noradrenergic nucleus located in the pons. The locus coeruleus is thought to be a center that alerts the brain to the possibility of danger when a threatening or novel stimulus is encountered. Panic anxiety is thought to be related to dysregulation of this center, leading to paroxysmal bursts of hyperactivity of functions driven by norepinephrine, that cannot be contained by other regulatory circuits in the brain. Dysregulation of the locus coeruleus may occur spontaneously, or it may become conditioned after repeated exposure to situations that stimulate it strongly. The latter mechanism may be important in PTSD, in which the patient reacts strongly to a situation that arouses great anxiety and then continues to react spontaneously after the situation changes.

An important braking mechanism on the locus coeruleus is the gamma aminobutyric acid (GABA) receptor complex, located on the noradrenergic neuron. When it interacts with its receptor, GABA causes chloride channels to open, increasing influx into the neuron of negatively charged ions. The resulting increase in net negative internal charge hyperpolarizes the locus coeruleus neuron, making it more difficult for it to discharge and therefore decreasing its activity in alerting the brain.

The GABA receptor is linked to a benzodiazepine receptor that interacts with benzodiazepine tranquilizers and theoretically with an as yet unidentified endogenous antianxiety ligand. Stimulation of the benzodiazepine receptor causes changes in the cell membrane that increase the affinity of the GABA receptor for GABA. As a result, chloride ion influx is greater in response to the same amount of GABA activity and the neuron becomes more resistant to depolarization than would be the case if the GABA receptor were stimulated by GABA alone (8). Substances that interfere with the action of the GABA-benzodiazepine-chloride ion channel complex impair the locus coeruleus control mechanism and cause intense generalized anxiety, while compounds that facilitate the action of the complex hyperpolarize locus coeruleus neurons and reduce the neuronal alerting response to any situation that is perceived as dangerous. These observations suggest that anxiety may be related to endogenous factors that block some aspect of the GABA mechanism in the locus coeruleus (7).

■ DIFFERENTIAL DIAGNOSIS

The first step in evaluating any anxious patient is to exclude illnesses (Table 1) and medications (Table 2) that cause anxiety. A common problem occurs when patients who have been taking CNS depressants become more anxious when they withdraw from the drug, forcing them to take even more of the medication, drug, or alcohol to prevent further withdrawal. It can be difficult to convince these patients that the substance is causing and not helping the anxiety.

A number of primary psychiatric disorders can be associated with anxiety that is so severe that it appears to be the primary problem. These include:

Organic mental syndromes. Delirious patients frequently become anxious, in part because their confusion is frightening to them and in part because the organic process affects the locus

TABLE 1. **Illnesses That May Cause Anxiety**

Cardiovascular
  Arteriosclerotic heart disease
  Paroxysmal tachycardias
  Subacute bacterial endocarditis

Endocrine/Metabolic
  Hypoglycemia
  Thyroid disease
  Parathyroid disease
  Cushing's syndrome
  Porphyria
  Hypokalemia
  Hyponatremia

Neurological
  Temporal lobe epilepsy
  Multiple sclerosis
  Organic mental syndrome of any cause
  Menière's disease

Tumors
  Pheochromocytoma
  Carcinoid
  Insulinoma

Pulmonary
  Hypoxemia
  Pulmonary embolism

Infectious
  Tuberculosis
  Brucellosis

TABLE 2. **Medications and Nonprescription Drugs That May Cause Anxiety**

CNS stimulants (e.g., amphetamine, cocaine)
Neuroleptics (akathisia)
Caffeine
Monosodium glutamate
Withdrawal from CNS depressants (e.g., alcohol, tranquilizers)
Any drug that clouds sensorium in hypervigilant patients

coeruleus and the limbic system. The differentiation between primary anxiety disorders and anxiety caused by an organic mental syndrome is crucial because most tranquilizers depress brain function and worsen organic mental syndromes (Table 3).

Psychosis. When a patient is blatantly psychotic, anxiety caused by psychological disorganization is easily recognized. Early in their course, however, the psychotic process in mania, psychotic depression, schizophrenia, and brief reactive psychoses may be overshadowed by severe anxiety that represents a reaction to losing control of basic mental functions. Careful questioning about hallucinations, delusions, sleep disturbances, and idiosyncratic ideas that are making the patient anxious usually uncovers the underlying disorder. Psychotic anxiety is treated with neuroleptics rather than antianxiety drugs.

■ TREATMENT

Before adding new treatments, it is essential to discontinue psychoactive substances that are taken to alleviate anxiety but

TABLE 3. **Anxiety and Organic Mental Syndromes**

Organic Mental Syndrome	Anxiety
Anxiety fluctuates and alternates with other emotions	Anxiety is constant, accompanied by brief bursts of stereotyped panic anxiety or varies with symbolically meaningful events
Mental status abnormalities are consistent (e.g., disorientation and impaired short-term memory with remote memory intact)	Inconsistent mental status abnormalities (e.g., long-term memory more impaired than recent memory)
Performance on mental status examination does not improve significantly with reassurance	Performance improves with reassurance
Symptoms worsen with CNS depressants	Symptoms improve temporarily with tranquilization
No reliable family history	Family history of anxiety or depression may be present

actually increase it. Caffeine should be completely discontinued; even "caffeine-free" coffee and cola may contain enough caffeine to be anxiogenic. If controlling medications and other substances and treating illnesses that could be aggravating anxiety does not resolve the problem, specific treatments should be added.

DRUG THERAPY OF ANXIETY

Six classes of medications are used to treat anxiety: cyclic antidepressants, MAOIs, benzodiazepines, buspirone, beta adrenergic blockers, and antihistamines (9–14).

INDICATIONS

Panic disorder
All cyclic antidepressants with the exception of bupropion (not yet released), and all MAOIs, ameliorate panic attacks. Some clinicians find that the MAOIs are more predictably beneficial. The same dose used to treat depression is prescribed for panic anxiety, and the same delay in onset of therapeutic effect frequently is encountered. Of the benzodiazepines, only alprazolam and clonazepam have been shown to be reliably effective for panic attacks. No other tranquilizer has been demonstrated to be useful in the usual doses.

Anticipatory anxiety
Not infrequently, subpanic and anticipatory anxiety associated with panic disorder abate when the panic attacks are successfully treated with antidepressants. Benzodiazepines may be helpful for residual anticipatory anxiety or avoidance if behavioral techniques alone are not sufficient.

Generalized anxiety
Benzodiazepines and buspirone are used to treat generalized anxiety. While some chronically anxious patients with limited psychological resources or unremitting situational problems may need long-term support of coping skills with an antianxiety drug, the anxiolytics are best suited for patients who:

- are anxious in response to a time-limited stress
- have responded to antianxiety drugs in the past

- will not need to take medication for more than a few months
- are not substance abusers
- are motivated
- view their anxiety as psychological
- feel better in the first few weeks of treatment

Addiction-prone patients with time limited anxiety

Because of the risk of dependence and abuse, benzodiazepines should be avoided whenever possible in patients with a history of alcoholism or other substance use disorder. When these patients have bona fide indications for a tranquilizer, buspirone or antihistamines are preferable.

Anxiety mixed with depression

Whenever anxiety and depression are mixed, an attempt should be made to use an antidepressant alone. Alprazolam, which is thought by some clinicians to have antidepressant properties, or buspirone, which does not seem to aggravate depression, may be the most logical antianxiety drugs when depressed anxious patients need adjunctive antianxiety treatment early in the course of therapy. Anxiety frequently resolves when the depression is treated adequately.

Phobias

When it is a complication of panic disorder, agoraphobia is treated with an antidepressant. Benzodiazepines may be used as adjunctive medications in the behavioral therapy of simple phobias. Social phobia has been treated with antidepressants and beta adrenergic blockers.

PTSD

Cyclic and MAOI antidepressants have been used to treat PTSD with variable success. To the extent that this disorder involves escalating reactivity to decreasing external stimulation by an actual trauma, kindling mechanisms may be involved (i.e., neurons that are repetitively stimulated become hypersensitive and eventually discharge autonomously). If this is a mechanism of PTSD, carbamazepine, an anticonvulsant that decreases kindling, might be helpful. Only informal studies of this hypothesis have been reported.

Stage fright

Stage fright, test anxiety, and some cases of anxiety associated with significant cardiovascular symptoms or tremor respond well to beta blockers, particularly propranolol, which is taken in anticipation of an episode of anxiety.

MECHANISMS OF ACTION

Antidepressants may reduce panic anxiety by normalizing activity of norepinephrine in hyperreactive locus coeruleus neurons. Another mechanism, which is more likely in drugs such as trazodone that increase brain serotonin levels, may be to strengthen systems that compensate elsewhere in the brain for excess locus coeruleus activity. All anxiolytics except buspirone act on the GABA receptor complex described earlier (5). Beta blockers that enter the brain, such as propranolol, probably have a central effect on brain beta receptors in addition to their peripheral action, while those that do not (e.g., atenolol) appear to decrease end organ responsiveness to sympathetic stimulation, thereby diminishing cardiovascular and motor responses that, when perceived by the patient, increase the sense of anxiety.

PREPARATIONS, DOSAGE, SIDE EFFECTS, AND INTERACTIONS

Anxious patients tend to be excessively sensitive to side effects of all medications because these patients are hypervigilant for the slightest malfunction within or outside themselves. It may also be that the nervous systems of anxious patients are hypersensitive to any perturbation, including changes induced by drugs.

ANTIDEPRESSANTS

Many heterocyclic antidepressants increase intrasynaptic norepinephrine, at least initially. Early elevations of noradrenergic activity in the locus coeruleus can cause such side effects as increased anxiety, jitteriness, tremor, tachycardia, sweating, and insomnia. When the overall action of the transmitter is eventually stabilized after a month or two, these side effects often wear off. Starting with low doses (e.g., 10 mg of imipramine) and raising the dose very gradually may minimize mental arousal and behavioral activation produced by antidepressants. Serotonergic antidepressants such as trazodone and phenelzine may be better tolerated by some patients.

BENZODIAZEPINES

Benzodiazepines (Table 4) are the standard treatment for situational and generalized anxiety. These medications are safe with respect to overdose and interactions and have a lower potential for abuse than previous generations of antidepressants such as bromides, barbiturates and propanediol carbamates (e.g., meprobamate).

Benzodiazepines are well absorbed orally, but with the exception of lorazepam, they have unpredictable availability after intramuscular administration. Most benzodiazepines are metabolized in the liver. Unlike the barbiturates and many other psychoactive drugs, they do not induce their own metabolism or the breakdown of other medications. With a few exceptions (e.g., lorazepam) the degradation of most benzodiazepines is inhibited by cimetidine and oral contraceptives.

Variable patterns of metabolism of benzodiazepines to active or inactive products result in a broad range of durations of action (Table 4). Despite half-lives of up to two days, benzodiazepines are usually given in divided doses to avoid peak serum concentrations that can cause excess sedation.

The most important adverse effects of benzodiazepines are sedation, tolerance, and abstinence syndromes. Paradoxical reactions such as anxiety, irritability, aggression, agitation, and insomnia can occur in children, the elderly, brain damaged patients, and chronically hypervigilant individuals. Fatal overdose is rare unless other CNS depressants are ingested at the same time.

Between 45% and 100% of patients using therapeutic doses of benzodiazepines for three months or more experience some form of abstinence syndrome (6). Even one dose of a benzodiazepine can produce rebound anxiety or insomnia. The risk of tolerance and/or withdrawal is significant in patients who take 40–60 mg/day of diazepam or its equivalent for a month or who take lower doses (e.g., 15 mg/day) for more than 8–12 months (17,18). Abstinence syndromes are more intense with shorter acting preparations such as lorazepam and alprazolam; withdrawal appears a week or two later and is more prolonged and

TABLE 4. **Commonly Used Antianxiety Drugs**

Class and Drug	Trade Name	Usual Daily Dose (mg)	Effect
Short-acting benzodiazepines[a]			
Lorazepam	Ativan	2–6	Intermediate
Oxazepam	Serax	45–100	Slow
Alprazolam	Xanax	1.5–6.0	Intermediate
Halazepam	Paxipam	20–120	Fast
Temazepam	Restoril	15–30	Intermediate
Triazolam	Halcion	0.125–0.5	Fast
Intermediate-acting benzodiazepines[b]			
Clonazepam	Klonipin	1.5–1.6	Slow
Long-acting benzodiazepines[c]			
Diazepam	Valium	2–40	Fastest
Chlordiazepoxide	Librium	10–100	Intermediate
Clorazepate	Tranxene	7.5–60	Fast
Prazepam	Centrax	10–60	Slowest
Flurazepam	Dalmane	15–30	Slow
Azospirodecanedione			
Busiprone	Buspar	5–40	Slow
Antihistamines			
Hydroxyzine	Atavax	100–200	Slow
Diphenhydramine	Benadryl	100–200	Slow
Beta-blockers			
Propranolol	Inderal	40–120	Slow
Atenolol	Tenormin	25–50	Slow

[a] Half-life 5–20 hrs.
[b] Half-life 20–40 hrs.
[c] Half-life 20–200 hrs.

attenuated with the longer acting benzodiazepines. Alprazolam and other benzodiazepines may not suppress each other's abstinence symptoms, so substituting one for the other may not prevent withdrawal. Subtle signs of benzodiazepine withdrawal have been reported six months to a year after the drug has been discontinued (16). Manifestations and management of withdrawal from benzodiazepines and other CNS depressants are discussed in Chapter 6.

BUSPIRONE

Buspirone (Table 4) is a new nonbenzodiazepine azospiro-decanedione antianxiety drug with the same indications as the benzodiazepines (19). It differs from the latter class of drugs in that it does not cause tolerance, abstinence syndromes, muscle relation, or sedation and does not raise the seizure threshold. Higher doses cause dysphoria, making addiction unlikely. Buspirone must be given regularly in divided doses, sometimes for as long as a month, before its antianxiety effect becomes manifest; as needed dosing therefore is usually not effective. Because buspirone does not cross-react with other CNS depressants and will not suppress withdrawal from these drugs, it cannot be directly substituted for them.

ANTIHISTAMINES

Hydroxyzine and diphenhydramine (Table 4) are sometimes used as antianxiety drugs and hypnotics for addiction-prone patients and the elderly. Antihistamines are not habituating but they are sedating and anticholinergic, and their antianxiety effect is unpredictable.

BETA ADRENERGIC BLOCKING AGENTS

A single dose of 10–40 mg of propranolol taken prior to performance can block stage fright and test anxiety. Propranolol and atenolol may diminish symptoms of sympathetic arousal associated with acute anxiety. Atenolol has been used to treat social phobia and to block adrenergic arousal produced by antidepressants.

SELECTION OF AN ANTIANXIETY DRUG

Benzodiazepines are selected according to the following guidelines (13, 14, 20, 21):

1. Shorter acting benzodiazepines and buspirone are better tolerated by elderly and brain damaged patients.

2. Benzodiazepines with simpler metabolic pathways, such as lorazepam and oxazepam, are theoretically better tolerated by patients with liver disease, although clinical problems with other benzodiazepines may be less common in these individuals than has generally been thought.
3. All benzodiazepines with the possible exception of alprazolam can aggravate depression.
4. Unlike most other benzodiazepines, alprazolam in doses as high as 6–12 mg/day is effective for panic disorder. Alprazolam is frequently better tolerated than antidepressants, but because of its short half-life it must be taken frequently—sometimes every two hours or so—or withdrawal symptoms appear between doses. No single dose should be larger than 1 mg. Even when the dose is decreased as slowly as by 0.25 mg per month, withdrawal anxiety can make it difficult to withdraw the drug. Alprazolam can be started along with an antidepressant in patients with panic disorder to produce rapid release and diminish activating symptoms of the antidepressant. Alprazolam is gradually withdrawn as soon as the antidepressant begins working.
5. Clonazepam is the only other benzodiazepine that has been found to be useful in panic disorder. It has a longer half-life than alprazolam, minimizing interdose withdrawal and severe difficulty withdrawing the drug. However, it is more sedating and is more likely to cause depression.
6. Barbiturates and related CNS depressants should not be used to treat any form of anxiety except certain abstinence syndromes described in Chapter 6. A few patients who have been taking these drugs for many years may find it difficult to discontinue them, but even these patients often can be very gradually switched to a benzodiazepine once a stable relationship with the physician has been established.

■ **PSYCHOLOGICAL AND BEHAVIORAL MANAGEMENT OF ANXIOUS PATIENTS**

Every clinician treating anxiety should be familiar with at least a few of the many effective approaches that are available. These include (3, 22):

REASSURANCE

Because anxious patients worry continually about how safe they are in the doctor's hands, the physician can expect to be questioned repeatedly about every drug and therapeutic maneuver. Some chronically anxious patients are extraordinarily well read, and it is often necessary to be intimately familiar with symptoms of anxiety and with drug actions and side effects in order to reassure that patient confidently and authoritatively. The physician's credibility can be increased by predicting the patient's feelings, for example, by asking whether he or she has become more dependent on others or more reluctant to leave home before the patient volunteers the information.

INTERVENTIONS BASED ON SPECIFIC ANXIETIES

It often is helpful to address specific forms of anxiety in physically ill patients who are anxious about some implication of the illness. For example, brief frequent visits by nursing and medical staff are helpful to patients with separation anxiety. Patients with separation anxiety or stranger anxiety should have unrestricted visits by familiar people and limited visits by people they do not know. The patient who is anxious about the prospect of becoming dependent should be reminded that it will only be necessary to be dependent until the illness resolves; excessive displays of concern that may stimulate dependency wishes should be avoided. Patients who are anxious about losing control should be given as much control as possible, for example by asking them when the next visit should be scheduled or when it makes sense to take medication. Patients who are concerned that an illness or operation will make them unattractive or unlovable should be reassured that they retain many important qualities.

EXPOSURE

By itself, graduated exposure to an anxiety-provoking situation may overcome a simple phobia. Adjunctive treatment with a benzodiazepine or with specialized relaxation techniques are added if necessary to help the patient associate relaxation instead of anxiety with feared objects and situations.

RELAXATION TECHNIQUES

Any technique that induces relaxation decreases anxiety because it is impossible to feel tense and relaxed at the same time. The goal of relaxation techniques is to teach patients to focus their attention on a state of relaxation and away from anxiety. Relaxation may be induced by hypnosis, biofeedback, progressively relaxing one muscle group after another, or first tensing and then relaxing different muscle groups. States of mind that are the opposite of anxiety such as control, safety, and comfort are suggested at the same time in order to help the patient experience as many feelings as possible that are incompatible with anxiety.

SYSTEMATIC DESENSITIZATION

Systematic desensitization is a specialized technique used to treat phobias. First, the patient writes down an "anxiety hierarchy" listing every situation in which anxiety is experienced, ranked in order from the least to the most anxiety provoking. Next, the patient uses a relaxation technique and pictures a scene of great comfort, safety, and control, say a beach with the spouse nearby. The patient then pictures the first situation on the anxiety hierarchy and signals the clinician at the moment that anxiety begins to appear. At this point the patient is instructed to return to the safe, relaxing scene until the anxiety is gone. When relaxation is complete again, the patient mentally returns once more to the phobic situation. By relaxing each time anxiety begins to appear, the patient learns to feel comfortable and in control instead of anxious in each situation in the anxiety hierarchy. "In vitro" desensitization in the office or hospital must be followed by "in vivo" desensitization, in which the patient actually enters each situation in the hierarchy. A familiar person is present and the patient uses self-hypnosis or another relaxation technique if anxiety begins to appear, leaving the situation if necessary to avoid anxiety. In this way, the habit of relaxation is transferred to actual phobic settings.

SUPPORT

People become anxious because intact defenses and coping skills that make them feel safe are overwhelmed by external stress, by the danger of internal conflicts or physiologically determined arousal, or because inadequate defenses cannot cope with stresses that are not inherently overwhelming. Defenses can be shored up to restore equilibrium by encouraging the patient to do whatever is usually helpful at difficult times; for example, exercise, mental activity, or group projects. Environmental supports should be mobilized and unnecessary stresses reduced. The most meaningful support for most people comes from an important relationship that is readily available, especially with significant others and the physician.

INSIGHT

People with longstanding generalized anxiety, or patients with ongoing anxiety related to a chronic illness, may benefit from exploration of the symbolic meaning of the illness or other stresses. It may be particularly helpful to become aware of the tendency to expect the worse and then magnify slightly adverse consequences while ignoring the greater weight of evidence that nothing bad has happened. Insight into emotional conflicts has not been shown to reduce panic anxiety.

DENIAL

Physically ill patients are likely to become more anxious if they are encouraged to think about the danger they are in or to look into the meaning of symbolic conflicts during the acute phase of the illness. Encouraging these patients not to pay too much attention to the implications of the situation, and giving them tasks to take their minds off an acute problem about which nothing can be done except wait for it to improve, is often the most helpful approach at this point.

FAMILY TREATMENT

Patients who are anxious in the setting of a significant relationship should be treated in the context of that relationship whenever possible. The family should be mobilized to help to reassure the acutely anxious patient. Spouses of agoraphobics and other patients who have been severely incapacitated by anxiety often find it difficult to adjust to the patient's ability to function without them after successful treatment. They may then need to be encouraged not to undercut the patient's progress (e.g., by accusing him or her of being "hooked" on medication or by repeatedly asking if the patient needs assistance).

■ WHAT IF THE PATIENT DOES NOT RESPOND?

If the patient is not faced with external stresses or profound inner weaknesses that cannot be resolved, the prognosis for treatment of anxiety is good. When the patient does not improve as expected, a few questions can usually uncover the cause of treatment resistance:

1. Is there an organic etiology that is being overlooked? The most frequently overlooked physical causes of anxiety are covert alcohol and tranquilizer abuse, continued use of caffeine, and thyroid disease.

2. Am I using antianxiety drugs correctly? Patients taking short acting benzodiazepines at night may experience rebound anxiety the next morning. If they do not take the tranquilizer frequently enough, they may also have withdrawal anxiety at various times during the day. Taking larger doses with the same frequency only increases the intensity of interdose withdrawal symptoms. A better approach is to give smaller doses more frequently or use a longer acting benzodiazepine.

3. Am I avoiding discussion of a major trauma? Some patients with PTSD have had such disturbing experiences that other people naturally do not want to hear about them, subtly changing the topic instead of encouraging the patient to talk about the trauma. Anxiety continues as a signal that the patient has not been heard.

4. Have I understood the patient's problem? The real reason why the patient is anxious may not have been understood. If the patient does not improve with one approach, it is a good idea to ask the patient whether another approach would make more sense. Marital and family problems that have not been addressed are common covert problems.

5. Is anxiety the patient's "ticket of admission" to the doctor's office? Continued complaints of anxiety may be the way the patient has of legitimizing continued contact with the medical system. The patient should be helped to determine whether there are other, more appropriate potential supports that are not being utilized. If not, the kind of ongoing care described in Chapter 4 may be necessary.

■ REFERENCES

1. Merikangas KR, Weissman MM: Epidemiology of anxiety disorders in adulthood, in Psychiatry. Edited by Michels R, Cavenar JO, Brodie HKH, et al. Philadelphia, J.B. Lippincott, 1987
2. Sheehan DV: Panic attacks and phobias. N Engl J Med 1982; 307:156–158
3. Williams J, Spitzer R (Eds): Psychotherapy Research. New York, Guilford, 1984
4. Torgensen S: Genetic factors in anxiety disorders. Arch Gen Psychiatry 1983; 40:1085–1089
5. Ashok R, Sheehan DV: Medical evaluation of panic attacks. J Clin Psychiatry 1987; 48:309–313
6. Guerrero-Figueroa R: Effects of yohimbine on CNS structures: neurophysiological and behavioral considerations. Psychopharmacologia 1972; 25:133–145
7. Squires RF, Braestrup C: Benzodiazepine receptors in rat brain. Nature 1977; 266:732–734
8. Ninan PT: Benzodiazepine receptor-mediated experimental "anxiety" in primates. Science 1982; 218:1332–1334
9. Zitrin CM: Treatment of agoraphobia with group exposure in vivo and imipramine. Arch Gen Psychiatry 1980; 37:63–72
10. Robinson DS: Panic attacks in outpatients with depression: response to antidepressant treatment. Psychopharmacol Bull 1985; 21: 562–567
11. Klein DF: Psychopharmacologic treatment of panic disorder. Psychopharmacologia 1984; 25:32–36
12. Shader RI, Greenblatt DJ: Some current treatment options for symptoms of anxiety. J Clin Psychiatry 1983; 44:21–29
13. Charney DS, Woods SW, Goodman WK, et al: Drug treatment of panic disorder: the comparative efficacy of imipramine, alprazolam and trazodone. J Clin Psychiatry 1986; 47:580–586

14. Baldessarini RJ: Chemotherapy in Psychiatry. Cambridge, MA, Harvard University Press, 1985

15. Meltzer HY, Flemming R, Robertson A: The effect of buspirone on prolactin and growth hormone secretion in man. Arch Gen Psychiatry 1983; 40:1099–1102

16. Busto U, Sellers EM, Narango CA, et al.: Withdrawal reaction after long-term therapeutic use of benzodiazepines. N Engl J Med 1986; 315:854–859

17. Rickles K: Long-term diazepam therapy and clinical outcome. JAMA 1983; 250:767–771

18. Lader M: Dependence on benzodiazepines. J Clin Psychiatry 1983; 44:121–127

19. Ayd F: Buspirone: a review. International Drug Therapy Newsletter 1984; 19:37–42

20. Pollack MH, Tesar GE, Rosenbaum JF, Spier A: Clonazepam in the treatment of panic disorder and agoraphobia: a one-year follow-up. J Clin Psychopharmacol 1986: 6:302–304

21. Greenblatt DJ, Shader RI, Abernethy DR: Current status of benzodiazepines. N Engl J Med 1983; 309:354–358

22. Spitzer RL, Klein DF (Eds): Evaluation and Treatment of Psychological Therapies. Baltimore, Johns Hopkins University Press, 1976

SLEEP DISORDERS 3

Each year, more than 10 million Americans consult a physician about a sleep problem, and more than one-half receive a sleeping pill (1). Sleep disorders are particularly common in the elderly. In addition to the 28% incidence of sleep apnea in this population, it takes older people longer to fall asleep, and they wake up more frequently during the night. If they remain in bed longer and take naps during the day, their total amount of sleep is the same as in younger individuals; but if they do not, they become sleep deprived. Sleep disturbances in the elderly therefore represent decreased ability to sleep, not a decreased need for sleep (2).

Although sleep disorders are second only to headaches as

complaints that patients bring to physicians, many doctors are not familiar with appropriate treatment techniques. For example, even though most hypnotics (sleeping pills) lose their effectiveness within a month, 75% of the time these medications are prescribed for at least four months (3). Even more surprising is the finding that one-third of patients who get a prescription for a hypnotic report that they were not having trouble sleeping in the first place.

■ SIGNS AND SYMPTOMS

People normally fall asleep within 20 minutes of going to bed and sleep for seven to eight hours. Four kinds of disturbances in the normal pattern may occur (4).

INSOMNIA

Insomnia is defined as decreased amount of sleep or a normal amount of sleep that is nonrestorative (not restful). Insomnia is diagnosed when it has been present at least three nights a week for at least a month and when functioning during the day is impaired. Daytime impairment may take the form of fatigue, irritability, decreased performance, difficulty concentrating, or depression.

HYPERSOMNIA

Hypersomnia has two forms. The first is excessive sleepiness or attacks of sleep during the day that are not in compensation for lost sleep at night. The second type of hypersomnia is difficulty waking up, with a prolonged transition to the awake state. The diagnosis of hypersomnia is made when it has been present every day for a month or periodically for longer periods of time, and when it impairs social or occupational functioning.

DISTURBANCES OF THE SLEEP–WAKE CYCLE

Mismatches between the endogenous sleep–wake cycle and environmental schedules that dictate when a person should fall asleep and wake up result in sleep starting and ending either earlier or later than it should. The result may be difficulty falling asleep when the patient is supposed to go to bed, with a tendency to sleep late or feel sleepy during the day, or feeling sleepy early in the evening and waking up too early in the morning.

PARASOMNIAS

Parasomnias are disturbances of aspects of sleep other than falling or staying asleep or alertness during the day such as motor activity and dreaming.

■ CATEGORIES OF SLEEP DISORDERS

Sleep disorders are categorized according to whether they are associated with insomnia, hypersomnia, a disrupted sleep–wake cycle, or parasomnias. Some sleep disorders produce more than one type of symptom; for example, insomnia plus hypersomnia.

DYSSOMNIAS

Dyssomnia is a global category that includes insomnias, hypersomnias, and sleep–wake schedule disorders.

INSOMNIAS (DISORDERS OF INITIATING AND MAINTAINING SLEEP, OR DIMS)

There are several categories of insomnia. Psychophysiologic insomnia occurs in response to stress. Insomnia related to another mental disorder is caused by a primary psychiatric disorder such as depression or anxiety. Insomnia related to a known organic factor is produced by a medical illness, a physical malfunction such as sleep apnea, a drug, or a medication. Primary insomnia has no obvious cause. In the short sleeper syndrome, the patient sleeps less than normal but is not tired or dysfunctional during the day.

HYPERSOMNIAS (DISORDERS OF EXCESSIVE SOMNOLENCE, OR DOES)

Like insomnia, hypersomnias are categorized according to whether they are primary or are related to another mental disorder or a known organic factor. The most common cause of hypersomnia is sleep apnea, which is described below.

NARCOLEPSY

Narcolepsy is a relatively infrequent (<1% of adults) but important cause of hypersomnia. In narcolepsy, rapid eye movement (REM) sleep intrudes into daytime experience and appears prematurely during nighttime sleep, resulting in characteristic manifestations:

Sleep attacks in which the patient suddenly falls asleep during the day. If allowed to sleep, the patient wakes up after 20–40 minutes feeling refreshed.

Cataplexy is weakness of all voluntary muscles' except the diaphragm and extraocular muscles, that is triggered by strong emotions and sexual arousal. The patient usually remains conscious but may fall asleep.

Sleep paralysis is paralysis of all muscles except the eye and respiratory muscles that occurs as the patient is falling asleep.

Hypnogogic hallucinations are complex, vivid hallucinations that occur just as the patient is falling asleep.

Sleep apnea or *nocturnal myoclonus* (described below) occur in one-third of narcoleptics.

SLEEP APNEA

Sleep apnea, which causes both insomnia and hypersomnia, is characterized by periods during sleep when the patient stops breathing for at least 10 seconds at least 30 times per night or 5 times per hour. As blood oxygen saturation falls, arousal mechanisms are stimulated and the patient wakes up. However, consciousness is usually not fully regained and the patient is confused and disoriented, sometimes wandering around or falling out of bed. Multiple awakenings deprive the patient of sleep, leading to daytime fatigue, depression, difficulty concentrating, headaches, impaired functioning, and a tendency to fall asleep. Central sleep apnea is caused by failure of brain respiratory centers. Obstructive sleep apnea is characterized by intermittent upper airway obstruction and usually is associated with loud snoring, terminating in an apneic episode that is often followed by gasping, choking, and thrashing before the patient awakens partially and starts breathing again.

NOCTURNAL MYOCLONUS

Brief jerking movements at the onset of sleep (hypnic jerks) are normal. In nocturnal myoclonus, repeated gross clonic jerks of the legs occur during sleep. These may wake the patient up, or they may reduce sleep efficiency without actual awakenings. Myoclonus may be present on one night but not another. Nocturnal myoclonus is found in 12% of insomniacs, 3.5% of hypersomnia patients and up to 42% of the elderly.

RESTLESS LEGS SYNDROME

This problem is characterized by uneasiness and restlessness in the legs when the patient lies down or rests, leading to a powerful urge to move the legs or to get up and walk around. Most patients with restless legs syndrome also have nocturnal myoclonus, but only a few patients with nocturnal myoclonus have restless legs syndrome.

SLEEP–WAKE SCHEDULE DISORDERS (DISORDERS OF THE SLEEP–WAKE SCHEDULE)

These disorders develop when a patient's circadian sleep–wake cycle is out of phase with the environment. In the advanced type the patient feels sleepy too early in the evening and wakes up too early in the morning. In the delayed type the patient does not feel sleepy at bedtime and then has trouble waking up the next morning. In the disorganized type of sleep–wake schedule disorder, the biological clock tells the patient to become sleepy and wake up at unpredictable times, so that a major sleep period is absent. The variable type is caused by changing times at which the patient must go to sleep and wake up, as occurs with frequent changes of work shift or time zone.

PARASOMNIAS

Parasomnias are a group of dysfunctions associated with various stages of sleep.

DREAM ANXIETY DISORDER (NIGHTMARES)

Nightmares occur during REM sleep, most of which occurs during the second half of the night. In dream anxiety disorders the patient wakes up during the latter part of the night with a vivid memory of a frightening dream that usually involves a threat to survival, security, or self-esteem. On awakening, the patient is immediately alert and oriented.

SLEEP TERROR DISORDER (NIGHT TERRORS, OR PAVOR NOCTURNUS)

Night terrors abruptly awaken the patient out of deep, nondreaming sleep during the first third of the night. The patient wakes with a scream in a state of dread and is confused, disoriented, and unresponsive to reassurance, with signs of autonomic arousal such as sweating and tachycardia.

SLEEPWALKING DISORDER (SOMNAMBULISM)

Like night terrors, somnambulism is a deep sleep (i.e., not associated with dreaming) parasomnia that occurs during the first third of the night. The patient walks around and is extremely difficult to wake up or communicate with. Shortly after awakening the patient shows no impaired function but is amnesic for the episode.

■ PRESENT ILLNESS

A careful history is the first step in distinguishing among the many different conditions that can disturb sleep (5). At a minimum, any patient with a complaint related to sleep should be evaluated for:

Duration of the problem. Insomnia lasting less than three weeks or occurring only infrequently is usually not clinically significant.

Stresses and conflicts. Patients who cannot sleep when they are in bed with a spouse or who feel sleepy whenever they are with a certain person usually have a conflict with the other person. Stress reduction is more useful than medications for people who cannot sleep because of psychosocial stresses.

Psychiatric symptoms. Depression and anxiety are common causes of insomnia, and sleep disorders may produce psychiatric symptoms during the day.

Medical illnesses. Painful illnesses often make it difficult to sleep. Specific medical conditions described below may be associated with dysregulated sleep.

Sleep setting. Is the bedroom noisy or too well lighted? Does the patient read, think about the day's events, or watch television before trying to fall asleep? Do discussions or arguments with the bed partner take place primarily at bedtime? Is there a problem in the relationship with the bed partner? Exactly what happens when the patient tries to go to sleep?

Sleep schedule. Does the patient go to bed and wake up at the same time each day? Has there been a recent trip or change in work schedule that has changed the patient's usual hours of sleep and awakening?

Behavior during sleep. Loud snoring, gasping, choking, thrashing, periodic cessation of breathing, or falling out of bed suggest sleep apnea. Gross movements of the legs may indicate nocturnal myoclonus or restless legs syndrome. Chest or stomach pain or a bad taste in the mouth may indicate gastroesophageal reflux. Wandering around at night suggests somnabulism if the patient is not disoriented after awakening and sleep apnea if the patient is disoriented. Awakening in fear during the first part of the night is more likely to be due to sleep terrors, especially if the patient is confused or aroused, while awakening during the second part of the night after a bad dream that the patient remembers usually indicates nightmares.

Functioning during the day. Patients who do not feel tired, sleepy, depressed, or confused during the day usually do not have clinically significant sleep disorders. Abruptly falling asleep during the day suggests narcolepsy, sleep apnea, or alveolar hypoventilation (Pickwickian syndrome). Weakness in the knees during excitement suggests narcolepsy.

Use of psychoactive substances. Medications and alcohol frequently are used to induce sleep, but they are more likely to disrupt it. Caffeine taken after 5 PM can make it difficult to get to sleep at night.

Sleep log. People are notoriously inaccurate in estimating the length and quality of their sleep retrospectively. A nightly record of all events related to sleep often clarifies important details that the patient does not remember later or dismisses as irrelevant.

History from bed partner. The bed partner often is aware of behaviors that the patient does not notice, especially signs of sleep apnea, jerking of muscles, and somnambulism. The bed partner should also be questioned about the patient's use of medications, drugs, alcohol, and caffeine and about whether he or she thinks that the patient is depressed or anxious.

Sleep recording. If there is no bed partner or if the bed partner's contribution to the history is not definitive, an all-night tape recording of the patient while asleep may reveal snoring, cessation of breathing, screaming, thrashing, or falling out of bed.

■ FAMILY HISTORY

A family history of depression or anxiety suggests that one of these disorders may be to blame for a sleep disorder in the patient. The non-REM parasomnias such as sleepwalking and night terrors are often familial, and narcolepsy probably has a genetic component (6).

■ ASSOCIATED PROBLEMS

When evaluating patients with sleep disorders it is important to consider other problems to which these patients may be prone.

ABUSE OF SEDATIVES AND ALCOHOL

People who have had trouble sleeping frequently use a variety of CNS depressants to get to sleep. Tolerance develops to the hypnotic effect, but abstinence symptoms occur whenever the blood level falls. As a result, the patient has to continue taking the medication to prevent withdrawal while obtaining little ongoing relief from the sleep disorder. In fact, many hypnotics disrupt sleep, and withdrawal from shorter acting drugs may make it impossible to get to sleep if they are taken too early in the evening, or may wake the patient at the middle or end of the night if they are taken closer to bedtime (7). The immediate effect of alcohol ingested at bedtime is to facilitate sleep onset; however, its short half-life leads to falling blood levels later in the night with withdrawal that wakes the patient up. The patient does not realize that alcohol is causing insomnia more than it is helping and continues drinking to get to sleep. Alcohol-induced sleep disorders may persist for months or even years after the patient stops drinking (8).

DOCTOR SHOPPING

Patients whose sleep disorders are not accurately diagnosed may consult physician after physician, obtaining a prescription for a different sleeping pill or tranquilizer from each of them. They may strenuously resist discontinuing these medications, even though they are still having trouble sleeping.

INCREASED MORTALITY

For unknown reasons, people who habitually sleep less than seven or more than eight hours a night have an increased mortality rate from a variety of illnesses (2). The greatest increase in mortality is in those who sleep more than the normal amount, especially if they are elderly. Artificially making a person sleep too much or too little has not been demonstrated to affect health or mortality (9).

■ LABORATORY FINDINGS

Sleep disorders that cannot be identified clearly by history or sleep records are definitively diagnosed in the sleep laboratory, where multiple functions are measured and the patient can be observed. Daytime recording also is performed in appropriate circumstances. Sleep laboratory evaluation is used to clarify the diagnosis in sleep apnea, narcolepsy, depression, sleep terrors, nocturnal myoclonus, restless legs syndrome, parasomnias, and impotence (6, 10).

POLYSOMNOGRAPHY

Polysomnography is an all-night recording of EEG, eye movements (electrooculogram, or EOG), and muscle tone (electromyogram, or EMG). Electrocardiogram (EKG), respiratory rate, blood pressure, oxygen saturation, esophageal pressure, penile circumference, and other physiologic parameters are monitored when appropriate. The abnormality that is uncovered depends on the disorder (e.g., cessation of breathing during sleep in sleep apnea, awakening during non-REM sleep in night terrors, and reduced REM latency in depression).

MULTIPLE SLEEP LATENCY TEST (MSLT)

People who sleep adequately at night do not fall asleep easily during the day. Those whose sleep is inadequate fall asleep rapidly if given an opportunity to nap. In the MSLT, the patient is given 20 minutes 4–5 times a day in which to nap. Patients with insomnia fall asleep within 5–10 minutes after starting the nap. Sleep apnea patients fall asleep within 3–5 minutes. The more severe the sleep disorder, the more likely the patient is to continue to fall asleep rapidly on each successive test, while patients with less severe disorders fall asleep rapidly during the first few but not all trials.

■ ETIOLOGY

Sleep disorders can best be understood by appreciating the structure of normal sleep and how it can be disturbed (11–13).

KINDS OF SLEEP

Sleep can be divided into REM and non-REM (NREM). There are three stages of NREM sleep. Stage 1 is a transition between sleep and wakefulness. Stage 2, which follows stage 1 within a few minutes, is manifested by characteristic EEG changes (sleep spindles and K complexes) that mark it as the first stage of definite sleep. Delta (slow wave) sleep is the restorative stage of sleep. Most slow wave or deep sleep occurs during the first part of the night.

Dreaming occurs during REM sleep, when the action of all voluntary muscles except those of respiration and the extraocular muscles is inhibited. Normally, the first REM cycle appears 70–90 minutes after sleep onset. REM then reappears every 90 minutes or so, lasting longer as the night goes on, as deep sleep becomes less frequent. Most people have 3–6 REM cycles per night.

The manifestations of narcolepsy are due to inappropriate appearance of REM during the day or before the first stage 2 cycle during sleep. Cataplexy is produced by development during the day of the descending inhibition of muscle tone that occurs during REM sleep. Sleep paralysis is caused by very premature onset of REM sleep and its associated motor paralysis, so that the patient is aware of being unable to move before consciousness is fully lost. Hypnogogic hallucinations are really REM sleep images that intrude into consciousness before the patient is fully asleep. Depression causes early onset of the first REM cycle during sleep, as well as increased REM sleep during the first half of the night, decreasing the amount of time available for restorative slow-wave sleep.

THE SLEEP–WAKE CYCLE

Cycles of sleep and wakefulness are driven by pacemakers in the brain, one that causes sleep and one that awakens the brain. The alerting or arousal system is stronger, so it does not require as much stimulation as the sleep onset system to become prominent. The balance between the sleep onset and arousal systems in the brain depends on interactions between a number of different neurotransmitters, especially serotonin, catecholamines, and acetylcholine.

Without any external cues, the human sleep–wake cycle is 24–28 hours long. However, it is normally synchronized (entrained) to the 24-hour cycle of important environmental cues (zeitgebers, or "time givers") such as light, dark, and activity schedules. The most potent zeitgeber for patients with abnormal sleep–wake cycles is the time at which the patient is required to wake up.

The sleep–wake cycle can be disrupted by internal changes in the sleep or waking pacemakers, as occurs in depression, or by lack of synchrony between these pacemakers and environmental zeitgebers. A common cause of the latter problem is entrainment of the sleep–wake cycle to a day–night cycle that is no longer appropriate; for example, because the patient has moved to a new time zone or work schedule.

STRESS

Stress and excitement commonly cause insomnia by stimulating the arousal system, which easily becomes predominant over the sleep-inducing system. Trying harder to fall asleep creates increased tension and conditions arousal to the setting in which the patient is supposed to fall asleep. As a result, the wakefulness center is automatically turned on whenever the patient goes to bed. This is why patients with insomnia can often sleep when they are away from their usual sleep setting.

Transient trouble sleeping associated with stress can become self-perpetuating if the patient sleeps late after a sleepless night caused by stress. The later wake-up time is a powerful zeitgeber that resets the circadian sleep rhythm, making it begin and end later. As a result, it becomes harder to go to sleep at the usual bedtime because the brain is not ready to fall asleep until later at night. If the patient feels tired enough to take a nap during the day, the artificial sleep and wake times induced by the nap further desynchronize sleep from environmental cycles and make it harder to fall asleep at the appropriate time at night.

■ DIFFERENTIAL DIAGNOSIS

Certain mental and physical conditions that are associated with difficulty sleeping can easily be confused with primary sleep disorders. These should be considered whenever a sleep related complaint is evaluated (5, 6, 12, 14).

DEPRESSION AND OTHER PSYCHIATRIC DISORDERS

Thirty-five percent of cases of insomnia and many instances of hypersomnia are caused by other psychiatric problems, especially depression. When typical signs, symptoms, past history, and family history are present, it is likely that these are the cause and not the result of the sleep disorder. Early psychotic decompensation that presents as trouble sleeping can be identified by asking about hallucinations and delusions. The sleep disturbance of dementia is due to confusion and disorientation at night (sundowning), while in delirium there may be an additional primary disturbance of the sleep–wake cycle. Careful mental status examination usually uncovers the real problem.

PAINFUL PHYSICAL ILLNESSES

Any illness that causes pain can make it difficult to sleep. Arthritis and other musculoskeletal problems are the most common offenders. Adequate pain control is more helpful than a hypnotic in these cases.

GASTROESOPHOGEAL REFLUX

In older patients, weakness of the lower esophogeal sphincter may result in reflux of gastric contents during sleep. The patient may awaken with chest pain or a sour taste in the mouth, or arousal may only be partial with no awareness of reflux. Multiple complete or partial awakenings lead to insomnia and/or hypersomnia. Esophogeal motility studies clarify the diagnosis in unclear cases.

SUBSTANCE ABUSE

Patients who abuse CNS depressants frequently develop sleep disturbances that may persist for a year or more after they become abstinent. Whether substance abuse is a primary cause or a complication of the sleep disorder, it must be treated if sleep is to be improved.

MALINGERING

Drug addicts may feign insomnia, hypersomnia, or narcolepsy in order to obtain stimulants and sleeping pills, especially barbiturates and related compounds. These individuals can usually be identified by demands for specific drugs and/or specific doses, visits to multiple physicians, claims that prescriptions have been lost, exaggerated, threatening, or changeable complaints, and a history of antisocial behavior.

SEIZURE DISORDERS

Temporal lobe epilepsy can produce automatic behavior during sleep that mimics somnambulism. Myoclonic epilepsy is typically associated with nocturnal myoclonus. However, epileptic symptoms usually occur during the day as well as at night.

■ TREATMENT

There are three components to the treatment of sleep disorders: sleep hygiene (management of the sleep environment), medications for sleep (hypnotics), and special therapies for specific disorders.

SLEEP HYGIENE

Many sleep disorders can be treated by making the environment conducive to sleep. Every patient who has difficulty sleeping should be advised to try the appropriate measures prior to taking a medication (5, 6, 15–17).

1. Keep the room quiet. Even occasional noises can disturb sleep. If extraneous noises cannot be controlled (e.g., in the hospital), earplugs or white noise machines may be helpful. Inpatients with trouble sleeping should be placed in the most quiet section of the ward.

2. Avoid making the room too hot. A warm room is comfortable, but ambient temperatures above 75°F. impair sleep.

3. Follow a regular bedtime ritual. New situations or activities can cause arousal and make it difficult to get to sleep.

4. Do not go to bed if not feeling sleepy. Staying in bed when the patient feels awake conditions arousal rather than drowsiness to the sleep setting. The patient then becomes alert instead of sleepy upon getting into bed each night.

5. Get out of bed if not asleep within 20 minutes. Trying harder to fall asleep strengthens the association between tension, restlessness, alertness, and being in bed. To avoid this problem, the patient should get out of bed and do something else for 20–30 minutes before returning to bed for another 20-minute trial of getting to sleep. For the same reason, the patient should not remain in bed after waking up in the morning.

6. Follow a rigid wake-up schedule. Even if the patient does not sleep for most of the night, it is important to awaken at the same time each morning. Since time of awakening is one of the most important zeitgebers that regulates the sleep–wake cycle, a regular wake-up time eventually will help to stabilize the time of sleep onset.

7. Do not use the bed for activities other than sleeping or sex. Reading, watching exciting television shows, and other activities stimulate arousal centers, which are more potent in producing wakefulness than brain sleep centers are in producing sleep. A few patients, however, find that reading or watching television makes them more relaxed and helps them get to sleep.

8. Schedule a time before bedtime to review the day's events. Patients who do not have a chance earlier in the evening to review the day's activities and concerns may become aroused when they think about these issues while attempting to go to sleep. It is better to schedule a few minutes away from bed for this activity to avoid associating alertness with bed.

9. Avoid daytime naps. Sleeping during the day further disrupts the sleep–wake cycle. No matter how tired the patient feels, a regular sleep pattern is more likely to be induced by remaining awake during the day and going to bed earlier that night. An important exception is the older patient whose sleep is intrinsically inefficient and needs additional sleep during the day.

10. Do not use caffeine after the early afternoon. Caffeine, with a half-life of 4–5 hours, can impair sleep if it is taken later in the day. Nicotine may also impair sleep.

11. Exercise during the day. Moderate daily exercise facilitates sleep at night. However, exercising strenuously shortly before bedtime produces arousal rather than sleepiness.

12. Use relaxation techniques. Biofeedback, hypnosis, relaxation exercises, and counting backward may counteract arousal that interferes with sleepiness at bedtime.

13. Consider a light snack at night. Hunger disturbs sleep. A light snack or a glass of warm milk, which contains the sleep-inducing substance tryptophan, prevents this problem. Heavy meals may interfere with sleep.

DRUG TREATMENT OF INSOMNIA

All hypnotics with the exception of antidepressants and antihistamines can produce dependence, withdrawal insomnia, and abnormal sleep. Once tolerance develops, increasing the dose does not improve sleep. Even when they are effective, the benefit of most hypnotics is more subjective than objective, since they do not increase time asleep by much more than 20–60 minutes, often without improving functioning during the day. To use hypnotic drugs effectively (7, 8, 18–20):

1. Withdraw any CNS depressants the patient is already taking. If the patient is sleeping badly while using hypnotics and alcohol, these substances are likely to be causing or contributing to the sleep disorder. Increased problems sleeping when CNS depressants are removed indicates withdrawal and not a need for more medication.

2. Use hypnotics for transient situational or stress-related insomnia. Hypnotics are most appropriately used for less than 2–4 weeks in situations in which the cause of insomnia is likely to resolve, such as acute illness, hospitalization, or change in time zone.

3. Offer sleeping pills prn to hospitalized patients. Hospitalized patients should not routinely be given hypnotics or they may respond to the expectation that they should have insomnia. In addition, they may become tolerant and then be unable to respond when they really need medication. They should be reassured that a sleeping pill is available if they begin to have trouble sleeping.

4. Use benzodiazepine hypnotics in most instances. A benzodiazepine sleeping pill (Table 1), or any other benzodiazepine (see Chapter 2, Table 4) with a similar duration of action (e.g., diazepam for flurazepam or oxazepam for temazepam) is the safest and most effective preparation available. Medication should be started in the lowest available dose and increased cautiously. Increasing the dose beyond the recommended maximum is not helpful.

5. Use only one benzodiazepine. If the patient is taking a benzodiazepine antianxiety drug during the day, the same medication should be given at night for sleep instead of adding a second benzodiazepine at bedtime.

6. Give hypnotics infrequently if they must be used chronically. To prevent habituation, tell the patient with chronic insomnia to take sleeping pills once or twice a week, and certainly no

TABLE 1. **Benzodiazepine Hypnotics**

Medication	Half-life (hrs)	Usual Adult Dose (mg)	Comments
Flurazepam (Dalmane)	≥48	15–30	Most appropriate for patients with anxiety during the day Accumulates after several days; can cause daytime sedation
Temazepam (Restoril)	8–12	15–30	Slowly absorbed: must be taken ½ hour before bedtime Best for patients who have difficulty staying asleep
Triazolam (Halcion)	1.7–3	0.125–0.5	Rapidly absorbed Best for patients with difficulty falling asleep May cause withdrawal anxiety in the morning Can cause transient global amnesia the next day

more frequently than 20 times per month. If the patient becomes tolerant, temporarily discontinue the medication to restore responsiveness. Many patients can stand a few sleepless nights if they know that a sleeping pill will help on other nights.

7. Caution about daytime sedation. Patients who must be alert during the day should not take sleeping pills at night, with the possible exception of triazolam.

8. Do not give hypnotics to patients with a history of heavy snoring until sleep apnea has been excluded. CNS depressants are dangerous to these patients because they increase the threshold for arousal and lower the level of oxygen saturation that develops before the patient begins to awaken.

9. Treat depressed patients with antidepressants. The appropriate hypnotic for a depressed patient with a sleep disorder is an antidepressant. Some depressed patients with hypersomnia respond better to MAOIs; if the medication is effective for depression the patient's sleep will improve, too, even though the medication is taken during the day.

10. Consider alternative treatments. Antihistamines (e.g., diphenhydramine 25–50 mg) are helpful to some elderly patients and do not cause tolerance or withdrawal. Tryptophan (1–5 mg) plus vitamin B_6 helps a few patients get to sleep. Low doses of sedating antidepressants (e.g., 10–50 mg of amitriptyline) may be helpful to some insomniacs who were hyperactive as children.

11. Avoid barbiturates, glutethimide, ethylchlorvynol, methylpryon, and related drugs. These drugs cause dependence and dangerous abstinence syndromes in addition to disturbing the structure of sleep (e.g., by severely suppressing REM sleep). Chloralhydrate is somewhat safer but has a narrower therapeutic index than the benzodiazepines.

TREATMENT APPROACHES FOR SPECIFIC SLEEP DISORDERS

Sleep disorders other than psychophysiologic (i.e., stress-related) insomnia, insomnia related to a psychiatric or physical disorder, and sleep–wake schedule disorders related to jet lag and work shift changes, require specialized treatments that are summarized in Table 2 (6, 12).

TABLE 2. **Treatment of Some Sleep Disorders**

Disorder	Effective Treatments	Comments
Sleep apnea	Weight loss Protriptyline Theophylline Acetazolamide Oxygen L-tryptophan Tracheotomy Reconstructive ENT surgery	CNS depressants aggravate sleep apnea and may be dangerous
Narcolepsy	Psychological support Group therapy Tricyclic antidepressants for cataplexy Stimulants for daytime sleepiness	Drug holidays often necessary to reduce tolerance to effective medications
Nocturnal myoclonus	Clonazepam Carbamazepine Diazepam	Antidepressants may aggravate or cause nocturnal myoclonus
Somnambulism	Low dose benzodiazepine Make environment safe	Benign long-term outcome if patient is not accidentally hurt
Night terrors	Benzodiazepines Tricyclic antidepressants Psychotherapy	Not necessarily a sign of psychopathology
Nightmares	Withdraw medications that can cause night- mares (e.g., anti- depressants) or give during the day Psychotherapy No drug treatment	Often a sign of psychological conflict or stress
Delayed and advanced sleep phase syndromes	Go to bed earlier each night until sleep onset coincides with appropriate bedtime	It is easier to turn the biological clock forward than backward

96

■ **REFERENCES**

1. Institute of Medicine: Report of a study: sleeping pills, insomnia and medical practice. Washington DC, U.S. National Academy of Sciences, 1979
2. Kripke DF, Simons RN, Garfinkel L, et al: Short and long sleep and sleeping pills: is increased mortality associated? Arch Gen Psychiatry 1979; 36:103–116
3. Tognoni G, Bellantuono C, Lader M (Eds): Epidemiological Impact of Psychotropic Drugs. Amsterdam, Elsevier, 1981
4. Association of Sleep Disorders Centers: Diagnostic Classification of Sleep and Arousal Disorders. Sleep 1979; 10(1)
5. Kripke DF, Gillin JC: Sleep disorders, in Psychiatry. Edited by Michels R, Cavenar JO, Brodie HKH, et al. Philadelphia, J.B. Lippincott, 1986
6. Hauri P: The Sleep Disorders, 2nd edition. Kalamazoo, MI, Upjohn Co., 1982
7. Kales A, Soldatos CR, Boxler EO, et al: Rebound insomnia and rebound anxiety: a review. Pharmacology 1983; 26:121–137
8. Adamson J, Burdick JA: Sleep of dry alcoholics. Arch Gen Psychiatry 1973; 28:146–149
9. Friedmann J, Globus G, Huntley A, et al: Performance and mood during and after gradual sleep reduction. Psychophysiology 1977; 14:245–250
10. Richardson GS, Carskadon MA, Flagg W, et al: Multiple sleep latency measurements in narcoleptic and control subjects. Electroencephalogr Clin Neurophysiol 1978; 45:621–627
11. Aschoff J, Hoffman K, Pohl H, et al: Reentrainment of circadian rhythms after phase shifts of the zeitgeber. Chronobiologia 1975; 2:23–78
12. Kales A, Kales JD: Sleep disorders: recent findings in the diagnosis and treatment of disturbed sleep. N Engl J Med 1974; 290:487–499
13. Hauri P, Hawkins DR: Alpha-delta sleep. Electroencephalogr Clin Neurophysiol 1973; 34:233–237
14. Orr WC, Robinson MG, Johnson LF: Acid clearing during sleep in patients with esophagitis and controls. Gastroenterology 1979; 76:1213
15. Bonnett MH, Webb WB, Barnard G: Effect of flurazepam, pentobarbital and caffeine on arousal threshold. Sleep 1979; 1:271–279
16. Bootzin RR, Nicasso PN: Behavioral treatments for insomnia, in Progress in Behavior Modification. Edited by Hersen M, Eisler R, Miller P. New York, Academic Press, 1978
17. Griffin SJ, Trinder J: Physical fitness, exercise and human sleep. Soc Psychophysiol Res 1978; 15:447–450

18. Hartmann E, Spinweaver CL: Sleep induced by L-tryptophan: effect of dosages within the normal dietary intake. J Nerv Ment Dis 1979; 167:497–499
19. Greenblatt DJ, Divoll M, Abernathy DR, et al: Benzodiazepine hypnotics: kinetic and therapeutic options. Sleep 1982; 5:S18–S27
20. Kales A, Kales JD, Bixler EO, et al: Effectiveness of hypnotic drugs with prolonged use. Clin Pharmacol Ther 1975; 18:356–363

SOMATIZATION AND SOMATOFORM DISORDERS

4

Somatization is the process by which an emotional problem is converted into a physical complaint. The result is a somatoform disorder, or a condition in which physical complaints are presumably caused by psychological factors. Most primary care practices are well supplied with somatoform disorders. Somatizing patients usually do not consult psychiatrists—and are offended when the possibility is suggested—because they consider their problems to be entirely in their bodies and not at all in their minds.

Anyone can become transiently preoccupied with bodily function following an acute, frightening illness in oneself or someone else, during times of stress, or when beginning an unfamiliar activity such as starting an exercise program for the first time or transferring to a new job. While these individuals are easily reassured, the complaints of somatizing patients return with renewed vigor no matter how strenuously they are told that there is nothing physically wrong.

■ SIGNS AND SYMPTOMS

The hallmark of somatoform disorders is one or more physical complaints for which there is no organic cause or that are out of proportion to any identifiable medical or surgical illness. These "functional" (psychogenic) symptoms (Table 1) are associated with characteristic attitudes toward the illness and with typical interactions with physicians and other health care providers.

THINKING

The term alexithymia has been applied to the thinking of somatizing patients. Literally meaning "absence of words for emotions," alexithymia occurs in people who think of themselves in purely physical terms (1, 2). It is not only that they avoid their feelings; they can barely conceive of emotions in any but bodily terms. When patients with alexithymia are asked how they felt after a stressful event, they describe a physical change such as an action (e.g., "I stayed busy") or a disturbance in functioning (e.g., "I had a headache"). They experience somatic manifestations of anxiety and depression such as insomnia, anorexia, or lightheadedness, but are not aware of the emotional component. Other people may see an obvious association between physical disturbances and strong emotions, but the connection is a mystery to the patient, who expresses only worry about being ill.

TABLE 1. **Characteristics of the Functional Somatic Complaint**

Symptom appears in association with a stress or emotion

Marked resemblance to symptoms experienced by an important person the patient has known

Dramatic descriptions of distress (e.g., "like a sharp stake in the eye") that go on at great length

Agonizing symptoms in the face of great tolerance for pain from operations and diagnostic procedures

Expectation of a magical cure

Denial or indignation when a psychological cause is suggested

Decreased intensity of distress when the patient is told that symptoms are organic

Worsening of old symptoms or appearance of new ones when the patient should be improving

EMOTIONS

Somatizing patients often become indignant and defensive when they are told that their symptoms are functional or when the seriousness of their complaints is minimized. They may become openly anxious, depressed, or psychologically disorganized when aggressive attempts are made to explore their feelings. Somatizers regularly evoke feelings of frustration, impotence, anger, and self-doubt in the physician, which is probably their way of nonverbally communicating feelings of which they are unaware.

BEHAVIOR

Somatizing patients are in frequent contact with physicians and medical facilities, as if they are attempting to demonstrate how ill they are (3). When they are reassured that the symptoms do not seem too serious, the complaints paradoxically increase. Conversely, when they are told that the problem is important and requires continued medical follow-up, physical symptoms stabilize or decrease. Somatizers see themselves as independent people even though they actually are very dependent on their physicians and families. Exquisitely sensitive to changes in the doctor–patient relationship, they react with their bodies rather than their minds with intensified physical symptoms when they are seen less frequently.

Patients with most somatoform disorders have a great affinity for medications, especially pain killers and tranquilizers. When a new medication is administered it has a positive placebo effect for a few weeks to a month or two, but it eventually stops working. Even though symptoms return, the patient is unwilling to give up the medication.

■ CATEGORIES OF SOMATOFORM DISORDERS

Although several types of somatoform disorder have been described, there are often more similarities than differences among somatizing patients encountered in clinical practice.

HYPOCHONDRIASIS

In hypochondriasis, functional physical complaints are accompanied by preoccupation with the belief or fear of having a serious medical illness.

SOMATIZATION DISORDER (BRIQUET'S SYNDROME)

Somatization disorder consists of a constellation of chronic multiple physical complaints or a belief of being sickly that begins before the age of 30 and causes the patient to consult a physician, take medications, or alter lifestyle. Typical symptoms include gastrointestinal distress (e.g., nausea, vomiting, abdominal pain, food intolerance), cardiorespiratory symptoms (e.g., dyspnea, palpitations, chest pain), neurological symptoms (e.g., amnesia, difficulty swallowing, double vision, weakness), sexual symptoms (e.g., burning in sexual organs, pain during intercourse), and female reproductive symptoms such as dysmenorrhea. The patient must have had at least 13 different complaints to warrant a diagnosis of somatization disorder.

SOMATOFORM PAIN DISORDER

This term is applied to patients whose only complaint is functional pain lasting at least six months.

CONVERSION DISORDER

A conversion symptom is a clearcut loss or alteration of physical function (e.g., paralysis or sensory loss) appearing in the context of a psychosocial stress or strong emotion (e.g., becoming angry) that stimulates unconscious desires or conflicts (e.g., about striking out at the object of the anger). The physical symptom solves the conflict by expressing it in disguised symbolic form and by removing the patient from the situation that stimulated the conflict. Many patients with this diagnosis are found to have an actual physical illness within five years.

BODY DYSMORPHIC DISORDER

This is a new diagnostic term that refers to excessive preoccupation with a slight or nonexistent physical anomaly in a patient who does not have delusions, anorexia nervosa, or transsexualism.

■ PRESENT ILLNESS

Somatization usually is apparent by early to middle adult life. Some patients do not recover as expected from an acute but minor illness or injury, while others develop gradually escalating functional complaints without any identifiable precipitant. Since most forms of primary somatization represent longstanding habitual approaches to dealing with emotions, patients who develop functional symptoms for the first time after the age of 50 are likely to have some other disorder.

■ PAST HISTORY

Many somatizing patients grew up under circumstances of emotional or physical deprivation, neglect, or abandonment. They may have had to play an inappropriate parental role because a parent was sick or absent, and it is not uncommon to learn that they left school at an early age in order to help support the family. They function as pseudoindependent caretakers of other people until a minor illness serves as the focus for somatization and regression from independent functioning.

■ FAMILY HISTORY

The familial transmission of somatoform disorders has not been formally studied. However, many somatizing patients have had a parent or other important figure, who, through actual illness or somatization, served as a role model for the use of physical incapacity as a means of interaction. Parents of the future somatizer tend to be unresponsive to their children's emotional needs while reacting readily to illness and injuries.

■ ASSOCIATED PROBLEMS

Certain problems that can complicate somatoform disorders may be indistinguishable at first glance from the functional illness. It is important to search actively for these conditions when stable somatic complaints increase, decrease, or change in quality for no apparent reason, when the patient suddenly decides that the symptoms are psychogenic, or when the patient does not respond as expected to the appropriate treatment.

PHYSICAL ILLNESS

When actual organ dysfunction develops in somatizers, frequently it is overshadowed and elaborated on by the somatization process, leading to complaints that appear functional. Concurrent organic disease is fairly common in longstanding somatizers because many patients are elderly, because medications and invasive procedures may create new pathology, and because somatization may be a reaction to the unconscious perception of an as yet unidentified illness. Somatization does not protect a patient from disease.

SUBSTANCE DEPENDENCE AND ABUSE

Physicians frequently prescribe tranquilizers, sleeping pills, and analgesics in an attempt to satisfy the somatizing patient's demand for immediate relief. The patient with several physicians may accumulate a variety of medications, at least some of them habituating. Expressions of physical distress then escalate in order to justify more prescriptions that can suppress withdrawal symptoms, to which the patient is as hypersensitive as he or she is to all bodily dysfunction.

COMPENSATION NEUROSIS

In the modern age of litigation and entitlement, it is not uncommon for somatizing patients to receive financial rewards for being ill. Potentially treatable somatoform disorders may become recalcitrant when the patient's livelihood depends on remaining impaired in order to receive continued workmen's compensation, disability, social security, or other benefits. The longer the patient relies on such payments for support, the less confidence he comes to have in his ability to support himself through other activities.

■ LABORATORY FINDINGS

Many somatizing patients request tests that they believe will finally uncover a demonstrable lesion that will officially brand them as ill. Agreeing to perform the more invasive investigations in order to placate the patient or prove that there is nothing really wrong often backfires, as the patient dismisses a normal result as a mistake or not definitive and overreacts to a minor abnormality or adverse reaction to the test. Laboratory tests should therefore only be performed when there is reason to suspect a specific medical disorder. There is no test for somatization.

■ COURSE

Conversion reactions are usually acute and time limited; when they persist after the stress that provoked them has resolved, a covert physical illness or another somatoform disorder should be suspected. Most other forms of somatization are chronic (4). They can be controlled by maintaining a stable doctor–patient relationship, but attempts to remove symptoms often aggravate the disorder. Some carefully selected chronically somatizing patients with supportive families, strong motivation to improve, and absence of significant secondary gain for disability can learn more adaptive ways of interacting and communicating emotion. Patients who receive large disability payments have a worse prognosis for recovery, especially if payment is contingent on remaining ill.

■ ETIOLOGY

One group of investigators has speculated that alexithymia may be related to abnormalities in limbic system connections that make it difficult to handle emotion (2). Whether or not this hypothesis will ever be proven, it is clear that alexithymia can also develop in a setting in which the expression of emotions is ignored or punished and no assistance is provided in learning how to distinguish bodily from emotional experience. Later in life, the patient is threatened by attempts to mobilize emotions that are experienced as physical rather than mental. Clinical experience supports several additional psychological dimensions of somatization (5–8).

DEPENDENCY CONFLICTS

Many somatizing patients grew up in families in which their emotional needs were misunderstood or ignored completely because important caretakers were sick, missing, or emotionally incapable of responding with sufficient warmth and interest. Continuing to feel the normal needs of childhood—needs such as the wish to be comforted, soothed, and cared for, to let someone else do the worrying—would be excrutiating, since there was no one to meet them. One solution to this dilemma is to pretend that the needs are not there; after all, it is impossible to feel deprived of something that one does not know is missing. By becoming a person who does not need anything, who meets other peoples' needs more than one's own, it is possible for a time to forget about one's own ungratified desires.

The only drawback to this solution is that human needs do not disappear if they are ignored: they merely go underground, continuing to exert an unconscious influence. And when the setting changes so that gratification is potentially available, it is impossible to meet needs efficiently if one does not know that they are there. The more a person ignores needs and feelings, the deeper the reservoir of ungratified desires becomes until a minor stress, illness, or injury makes a desperate search for a caretaker appear to be something that the patient is forced to do by virtue of having a physical problem that clearly requires attention. By this time, emotional needs have become insatiable, but the patient has never learned how to ask directly to get them met.

SICK ROLE

Western society frowns on people who openly ask others to gratify them. However, when people become ill, we excuse them from their usual responsibilities and encourage them to take it easy and let other people do the work for them. Such culturally sanctioned benefits are included in the sick role, a set of clearly defined rewards and responsibilities that apply to anyone who is ill. The sick role is conferred upon a person—who then acquires the title of "patient"—by a physician in making a diagnosis. In return for being cared for, made comfortable, made the center of a certain amount of attention, and relieved of the demands and responsibilities of other social roles, the patient implicitly agrees to seek treatment, follow the physician's advice, and attempt to get well.

The sick role provides a setting that can legitimize dependency, but only to those who are labeled as ill by the medical system. The physician, therefore, plays a crucial role in certifying that the patient who needs to be physically ill in order to meet important needs is sick enough to deserve entry into the sick role. The physician is also crucial in actually ministering to the patient's needs in the context of the sick role. A student has the same power as a physician to the patient who sees everyone in a white coat as having the authority to convey the sick role or take it away, to offer sustenance or refuse it. The somatizing patient's demand to be considered "really" ill therefore represents a demand to be entitled to the sick role.

There is an important conflict for the patient for whom the sick role is an appealing solution to the problem of how to meet dependency needs without becoming aware of them in a setting that feels legitimate. The patient must seek and cooperate with medical care, but if the illness is actually removed the sick role will be withdrawn. Since the patient has never learned other ways of meeting needs, this would threaten the only reliable gratification it has ever been possible to obtain. The patient's solution to the conflict is to try each therapy that the doctor recommends in order to comply with the requirement to seek treatment, but to covertly defeat the intended cure in order to remain in the sick role.

SYMBOLIC PARENTING, HOSTILITY, AND GUILT

In legitimizing the somatizing patient's needs and then actually meeting them, the physician is functioning as a parent figure, permitting the patient to be dependent in ways that the patient's real parents were unable to gratify. The parental stand-in feels good, but the patient also inevitably becomes angry because the physician can never be the kind of perfect caregiver that the patient might hope for in a parental surrogate: taking care of a sick adult is only a dilute substitute for inadequate parenting earlier in life. In addition, the patient is reminded of anger at the original inadequate parents, anger that, like other emotions, has been kept out of awareness. Since openly expressing hostility might result in retaliation by the physician (as it did from the parents), it is expressed covertly by continuing to be symptomatic, and by frustrating the doctor's attempts to resolve the illness and get the patient out of the sick role. At the same time, physical suffering is a punishment for hostility that is no less potent because it is outside of awareness.

SECONDARY GAIN

Secondary gain is any concrete benefit that accrues as a result of being sick. One obvious secondary gain is money. Equally important is the opportunity to avoid situations that are unpleasant and to excuse failure to live up to one's potential by saying "I would have been much more successful if not for this illness." Physical distress can be an important means of making others solicitous, keeping them from leaving, or frustrating and upsetting them if the patient feels incapable of having an impact in any other way. Secondary gain is never the sole cause of somatoform disorders, but it may become a powerful motivator for continued somatization.

■ DIFFERENTIAL DIAGNOSIS

Disorders in which functional somatic complaints are only one manifestation of a more generalized disturbance must be distinguished from somatoform disorders, in which somatization is the core process (9, 10).

DEPRESSION

Depressed patients often have vegetative symptoms or functional complaints such as headache and backache. Their dependency, self-preoccupation, social incompetence, and covert hostility also are reminiscent of the psychology of somatization. In clearcut cases it is often possible to distinguish between the two (see Chapter 1, Table 8), but it is not always obvious whether longstanding somatic complaints are due to chronic depression or a primary somatoform disorder, especially hypochondriasis. When the diagnosis is at all in doubt, a trial of an antidepressant often clarifies the situation. Functional complaints that are symptoms of depression resolve and the patient becomes more assertive and effective. Primary somatization may improve transiently, but symptoms return when the patient becomes threatened by loss of the sick role and demands to function more effectively.

ANXIETY

Hypervigilance to minor bodily dysfunction, fears of having some terrible illness, dependency, and chronic physical symptoms of hyperventilation and autonomic arousal may make anxious patients resemble those with somatoform disorders, especially when the somatizing patient expresses anxiety about the symptoms. Treatment of the primary anxiety disorder completely resolves somatization secondary to anxiety, while the somatoform disorder improves briefly and then relapses.

ORGANIC MENTAL DISORDERS

Some demented patients distract themselves from a threatening primary disturbance of mental capability by directing their attention to minor bodily disturbances. Vague physical complaints may overshadow signs of the organic mental disorder if it is subtle, especially when the patient keeps insisting that the real problem is, say, a headache or backache. Functional complaints associated with organic brain disease are more changeable and inconsistent, and demands to be considered ill are less prominent than they are in primary somatoform disorders. The differential diagnosis is confirmed by careful mental status testing, which reveals typical disturbances of attention, concentration, and short-term memory. Both disorders coexist when somatizing patients develop organic mental syndromes from adverse drug reactions or interactions.

SCHIZOPHRENIA

Chronically psychotic patients may have delusions of having a serious illness that mimics hypochondriasis or somatic hallucinations that produce odd functional physical complaints. In patients who are in the prodromal or residual phase, typical disturbances of thinking may not be obvious until the patient is asked about idiosyncratic ideas about the nature of the illness and a mental status examination is performed. For example, a patient with schizophrenia may seem like any other somatizing patient until being questioned about the cause of the illness, when he or she reveals that the illness is caused by a ray from space.

MALINGERING

Malingering is the conscious simulation of disease for the sole purpose of obtaining significant secondary gain such as money, drugs, or escape from legal consequences. Malingering is almost always found in people with severe personality disorders (especially antisocial personality disorder) and those who are under severe stress (e.g., in the military). Treatment involves refusing to supply any reward whatsoever for the patient's illness. Factors that differentiate malingering from the more complex and unconscious processes of somatization are summarized in Table 2.

MUNCHAUSEN'S SYNDROME (FACTITIOUS DISORDER WITH PHYSICAL SYMPTOMS)

Like malingering, Munchausen's syndrome is characterized by conscious, purposeful simulation of disease. The patient may pretend to have physical symptoms or may even produce actual pathology through self-injury. However, the only goals in the factitious disorder appears to be to enter the sick role and deceive and humiliate the physician. The patient with a factitious disorder is distinguished by dramatic, changeable, unlikely symptoms that necessitate hospitalization or emergency treatment, use of pseudonyms, few visitors, and abrupt departure when the patient is confronted or a psychiatrist is called.

TABLE 2. Malingering and Somatoform Disorders

Malingering	Somatization
Patient is aware of simulating illness	Symptoms are not consciously produced but are unconscious solutions to complicated conflicts
Symptoms result in obvious significant gain	Secondary gain is only one aspect of the picture and involves interpersonal gain (e.g., meeting dependency needs) more than financial or legal gain
Past history of antisocial behavior and/or drug addiction	No past history of antisocial behavior
Personality disorder, especially antisocial or borderline personality	Somatization is a way of life but other signs of personality disorder are not as prominent
Patient becomes threatening when confronted and then abruptly leaves the hospital, emergency room, or clinic	Patient is indignant or anxious when psychological cause is suggested but becomes more dependent

■ TREATMENT

Most somatoform disorders are managed rather than cured. If the somatizing patient's need to be considered ill is accepted, it is possible to minimize the amount of suffering that must be demonstrated in order to be reassured of continued access to the sick role. Conversely, attempts to prove that the patient is not really ill result in an escalation of symptoms (7, 10–14).

DRUG THERAPY OF SOMATOFORM DISORDERS

Although there is no specific medication for somatization, it is the rule to encounter a somatoform disorder in which medications of one kind or another must be managed. Medicines are more important as tangible proof that the illness is sufficiently serious to warrant a physical treatment than for any pharmacological action. In addition, taking pills becomes the focus of a patient's day and forces continued visits to the doctor in order to refill the medication. Adverse consequences of medication can be minimized by following these guidelines:

1. *Avoid drugs that produce addiction, dependence, abstinence syndromes, and irreversible side effects* such as barbiturates, narcotics, and neuroleptics. It is easier not to start these medications than it is to discontinue them once the patient has become attached to them. Even severely somatizing patients usually accede to the physician's desire to protect them from long-term harm so long as the issue is discussed openly and a safer drug is substituted.

2. *Do not start a drug that does not have a clear-cut medical indication or that could not be continued indefinitely.* The safest medications are water-soluble vitamins, antihistamines, nonsteroidal anti-inflammatory drugs, amino acids, and, if necessary, benzodiazepines. These medications should all be prescribed with the same ritual as any other medication to indicate that the physician takes them seriously.

3. *Do not attempt to discontinue too rapidly medications that a new patient has been taking for a long time unless the drug presents an immediate risk.* It will be easier to withdraw the medication when a stable doctor–patient relationship has been established and the patient feels that giving up the medication will not mean giving up the doctor.

4. *Do not accede to demands for dangerous medication.* Occasionally, a somatizing patient begins treatment with a demand for a dangerous medication that is not medically indicated. Agreeing to such therapy even temporarily sets the stage for a doctor–patient relationship that is likely to be harmful to both parties. If the patient cannot accept a safer substitute, it is better not to begin treatment in the first place.

5. *Change to a similar medication when one drug loses its effectiveness.* It is tempting to increase the dose or strength of a medication when the patient seems to become tolerant. However, the reason that the medication has stopped working is more likely to be psychological than physiologic. A new medication may reassure the patient of the physician's continued interest and reopen the door to the sick role. Since the meaning of the medication is

more important than its pharmacology, the least noxious substitute should be used.

6. When analgesics are required, give them regularly. An "as needed" schedule makes the patient think about pain constantly in order to decide when it is severe enough to justify asking for the next dose, strengthening the association between symptoms, medications, and contact with doctors and nurses. In addition, if blood levels are not constant enough to suppress pain continually, higher doses may be needed as pain intensifies between doses.

7. Consider a trial of an antidepressant. Since it can be difficult if not impossible to distinguish chronic depression from a primary somatoform disorder, a diagnostic trial of an antidepressant is appropriate if there is no contraindication. Patients do not become physically or psychologically dependent on these drugs.

■ MANAGEMENT

Principles of management of somatizing patients are based on their ongoing need for sanctioned caretaking and their tendency to express problems of the mind in the language of the body:

1. See the patient regularly. If the patient is assured of ongoing access to a physician, it will become less necessary to use physical symptoms as a "ticket of admission" to the medical system. Somatizing patients should be accepted into outpatient treatment only with the expectation that they will need to be seen indefinitely. The more confident the patient is of the physician's continued availability, the less frequent the visits need to be. Initially, the patient might be seen once every 2–6 weeks for 15–30 minutes. As treatment proceeds, visits can be scheduled as infrequently as once or twice a year for 10 minutes or so.

2. Accept the patient's need to be considered ill. The patient should be told that even if symptoms improve considerably, the illness will probably always be present. Promise understanding and support but not relief, as this is as much of a threat as a reward.

3. Do not make contacts with the physician contingent on

somatic complaints. If remaining in the medical system depends on demonstrating illness, the patient will do so. If the patient knows that the doctor–patient relationship will continue even if the patient feels well, the use of symptoms as a means of ensuring access to the doctor will decrease.

4. *Do not prolong contacts with the patient in response to increased symptoms.* The patient should be told in advance how long visits will last. Visits should end promptly so that the patient will not learn to control the doctor's time with the illness.

5. *Set a discharge date in advance for inpatients.* Somatizing patients require hospitalization when they respond to psychosocial crises or changes in the relationship with the primary physician by reporting increased symptoms, when detoxification is required, or when a coexisting medical illness must be evaluated. Whenever it is medically feasible, a rapid discharge date should be agreed upon in advance. The goal of hospitalization should be to achieve a particular limited outcome (usually to stabilize medication or assure the patient of continued follow-up) and not necessarily to remove or reduce symptoms. Remaining in the hospital for too long may be so gratifying that it becomes very difficult to arrange discharge.

6. *Allow the patient to structure the content of discussions.* An open-ended question such as "how have you been feeling?" usually is sufficient. It is important not to become involved in prolonged speculations about the illness or arguments about whether the patient really is ill. Any comment by the patient about emotions should receive a more interested response, but it is necessary to be prepared to listen to physical symptoms without promising to do anything definitive about them.

7. *Minimize secondary gain.* If the patient is being paid for the illness, improvement is likely to be financially as well as emotionally threatening. Disability claims and litigation should therefore be settled prior to deciding on the goals of treatment. The family should be helped to avoid reorganizing their lives around the patient's illness, and be encouraged gradually to increase their demands that the patient function more effectively as a family member regardless of how he or she is feeling.

8. *Teach the patient to express emotions in words.* When the patient describes a situation in which a strong emotion such as anger should have been experienced but pain or some other physical sensation was felt instead, ask, "Were you angry, too?" If the patient responds that anger did not cause the pain, point out that anger and pain can be two different states that may or may not have anything to do with each other, but both are important to doctors who wish to treat the whole patient. General statements about important conflicts—for example, "There's nothing shameful about getting a little help from time to time"—may help the patient to begin very gradually to recognize concerns that feel too humiliating or overwhelming to be admitted to all at once.

9. Control strong reactions to the patient. Patients who assert a claim to the sick role but covertly refuse to cooperate with attempts to help them leave it frequently arouse strong feelings in the doctor. In response, it is common for physicians to forget appointments, vigorously attempt to prove that the patient is not really ill, tell the patient not to return unless symptoms become worse, or behave with excessive hostility or solicitude. Such impulses provide information about emotions that the patient is communicating nonverbally. Consulting with someone else can be very helpful in gaining control over and understanding the meaning of reactions to a patient.

10. Remain alert for intercurrent medical illnesses. Changes in the patient's symptoms that cannot be explained by new stresses or unavailability of the physician may mean that the patient is expressing a new medical problem in characteristic ways that make it appear to be more of the original functional complaint.

■ REFERENCES

1. Krystal H: Alexithymia and psychotherapy. Am J Psychiatry 1979; 33:17–31
2. Nemiah JC, Sifneos PE: Psychosomatic illness: a problem in communication. Psychother Psychosom 1970; 18:154–160
3. Mechanic D: The concept of illness behaviors. J Chronic Dis 1962; 15:189–194
4. Strain JJ, Grossman S (Eds): Psychological Care of the Medically Ill. New York, Appleton, 1976
5. Fann WE, Sussex JN: Late effects of early dependency need deprivation: the meal ticket syndrome. Br J Psychiatry 1976; 128:262–268
6. Twaddle AC: The concept of the sick role and illness behavior. Adv Psychosom Med 1972; 162–179

7. Engel GL: "Psychogenic" pain and the pain-prone patient. Am J Med 1959; 26:899–918
8. Ford CV: The Somatizing Disorders. New York, Elsevier, 1983
9. Drossman DA: The problem patient. Ann Intern Med 1978; 88:366–372
10. Dubovsky SL, Weissberg MP: Clinical Psychiatry in Primary Care, 3rd edition. Baltimore, Williams & Wilkins, 1986
11. Groves JE: Taking care of the hateful patient. N Engl J Med 1978; 298:883–887
12. Dubovsky SL: Psychotherapeutics in Primary Care. New York, Grune and Stratton, 1981
13. Neill JR, Sandifer MG: The clinical approach to alexithymia: a review. Psychosomatics 1982; 23:1223–31
14. Certcov D, Calvo J: The problem of psychotherapy in psychosomatic medicine. Psychosomatics 1973; 14:142–146

5 ORGANIC MENTAL SYNDROMES

Organic mental syndromes are changes in behavior, thinking, and emotional expression that are caused by an organic factor directly or indirectly affecting the brain. In a medical setting, particularly in the hospital, organic mental syndromes are much more common than any other psychiatric disturbance. It has been estimated that one-third to one-half of elderly patients become delirious during a medical hospitalization, and on some acute services the incidence of organic mental syndromes approximates 100% (1). Any personality change, psychosis, or behavioral disturbance in a medical or surgical patient should be considered an organic mental syndrome (OMS) until proven otherwise.

Organic mental syndromes, along with other major psychiatric disorders, are diagnosed by a systematic examination of mental functioning known as the mental status examination (MSE). The MSE is performed by observing and eliciting information about the status of five facets of psychological functioning. MSE findings in organic mental syndromes are summarized in Table 1 (2–4).

1. Appearance, attitude, behavior. Is the patient cooperative or uncooperative, friendly or belligerent, withdrawn or hyperac-

TABLE 1. **Mental Status Findings in Diffuse Organic Mental Syndromes**

Function	Findings
Appearance and manner	Fluctuating signs and symptoms
	Worse at night and in new surroundings
	Disheveled
	Confused
	Awareness varies from somnolent to hypervigilant
Speech	Incoherent
	Rambling
	Patient loses track of thoughts
	Dysarthric
	Dysphasic
Affect	Labile
	Shallow
Thought	Changeable delusions involving physicians and everyday events
	Impulsive suicidal or assaultive ideas
	Decreased foresight and impulse control
	Concrete, inflexible thinking
Sensorium	
orientation	Disorientation to time and place
memory	Impaired short-term memory
serial subtractions	Forgetting, confabulation, perseveration
digit repetition	Intact
constructional ability	Constructional and ideomotor apraxia
topographical memory	Getting lost; inability to identify directions
motor tasks	Difficulty starting and stopping; perseveration
proverbs and similarities	Concrete

tive, alert or confused? Are symptoms stable, or do they fluctuate in a predictable or unpredictable manner?

2. Speech and mental activity. Is speech logical and coherent or disorganized and incoherent? Is there any evidence of dysphasia, dysarthria, or words that the patient seems to be making up (neologisms)? Is the rate of speech fast or slow? Can the connections between ideas be followed easily or does the patient seem to be using an idiosyncratic form of logic?

3. Affect and mood. Is the patient's affect (outward expression of emotion at a particular moment) consistent with mood (enduring feeling tone as reported by the patient)? Is affect labile (unpredictably changeable) or shallow (lacking real emotional force and difficult to empathize with)? Is the patient sad, anxious, angry, or apathetic?

4. Thought content. Does the patient reveal any special preoccupations such as delusions, obsessions, phobias, suicidal, or homicidal ideas? Are these ideas stable and consistent, or do they vary from examination to examination? Are delusions systematized (complex) or concrete? Do they concern everyday events or are they highly implausible?

5. Sensorium. This segment of the MSE involves direct examination of various aspects of cerebral function:

• *Orientation.* The patient is asked the exact location (e.g., name of the ward and hospital or office address), day, date and time. Estimating the passage of a minute by counting to 60 or guessing the duration of the interview tests for subtle disorientation to time.

• *Memory.* Short-term memory is tested by asking the patient to remember three complex items for five minutes and by asking about recent events (e.g., what the patient had for lunch) that can be verified. Remote memory is tested by asking the patient about verifiable aspects of the history and by having the patient name the presidents in reverse order.

• *Attention.* Attention may be tested formally by asking the patient to repeat back in the same and in reverse order a series of random numbers (digit span).

• *Serial subtractions.* Serial subtraction of 7 from 100, 3 from 50, or counting backward from 50 by 1 test attention and short-term memory. The correctness of the subtractions is less relevant than whether the patient forgets his place, repeats previous answers (perseverates) or makes up answers (confabulates). Attention and short-term memory also can be tested by asking the patient to spell the word "world" backward.

• *New learning.* The ability to learn unfamiliar information requires intact attention, immediate recall, and recent memory. These functions can be tested by asking the patient to repeat back a complex phrase or sentence such as the Babcock sentence ("What this nation needs to be rich and strong is a safe, secure supply of wood"). Most people can learn the Babcock sentence within four trials.

• *Constructional ability.* Copying figures and drawing figures on command tests parietal lobe function.

• *Topographical memory.* Identifying directions to familiar places and locating major cities on a rough map depends on the intactness of the nondominant hemisphere.

• *Repetitive motor tasks.* Difficulty starting and stopping tasks such as repeatedly clapping the fist, edge, and palm of the hand against the opposite palm suggests frontal lobe dysfunction, as does perseveration of a previous response (e.g., continuing to clap the palm instead of moving on to the edge).

• *Interpretation of proverbs and similarities.* Describing the meaning of common sayings and the similarities between different objects tests the ability to conceptualize and think abstractly. The patient should be told to give the most general meaning of proverbs as they apply to all people, or to think of the broadest similarity between objects, such as a table and a chair. If the wrong answer is offered the patient should be told the correct interpretation at least once to ensure that the task has been understood. Concrete answers (e.g., "people who live in glass houses shouldn't throw stones" means "they'll break the glass") is seen in organic mental syndromes, schizophrenia, and low intelligence and education. Bizarre interpretations (e.g., "an apple is like an orange because they both squeeze the earth") suggest schizophrenia.

■ SIGNS AND SYMPTOMS

The manifestations of organic mental syndromes can be divided into primary and secondary disturbances. Primary manifestations reflect actual disturbances of brain function. Secondary disturbances are reactions to the primary disturbance that may overshadow it.

PRIMARY DISTURBANCES

Depending on the acuteness of the disorder, its etiology, and the region(s) of the brain that are affected, primary manifestations of disturbed brain function may include some or all of the following (5, 6):

Clouded consciousness. Decreased clarity of awareness of the environment is more common in acute organic mental syndromes.

Impaired attention. Difficulty paying attention and a wandering mental focus are seen in many organic mental syndromes.

Disorientation. Orientation to time is affected first, followed by orientation to place. Disorientation to person (i.e., not remembering who one is) is rare in organically induced conditions unless the patient has a very severe loss of memory.

Memory loss. Short-term (recent) memory is lost before remote memory. Immediate memory (e.g., ability to repeat back digits forward and backward) may be retained in the face of loss of recent memory of organic etiology, but loss of remote memory without significant loss of short-term memory usually is psychogenic.

Loss of higher intellectual functions. Thinking in diffuse organic mental syndromes is concrete, slow, and disorganized. Diminished ability to learn new and complex information leads to intolerance of change, a preference for the familiar, and intellectual rigidity.

Poor judgment. Impaired intellect, foresight, and impulse control make it difficult to anticipate the consequences of one's actions, refrain from impulsive behavior, or appropriately modulate social behavior.

Disturbances of the sleep–wake cycle. Delirious patients are most likely to exhibit sleepiness during the day, hypervigilance at night, and random alternations of alertness and drowsiness.

Focal cortical signs. A disorder that diffusely affects the brain or that is localized to one region of the cortex may produce signs of cortical dysfunction such as dysphasia and apraxia. Frontal lobe dysfunction may produce perseveration and difficulty initiating and stopping complex motor tasks.

Fluctuating symptoms. Unpredictable fluctuation of all symptoms is characteristic of acute organic mental syndromes and may be present in chronic syndromes. Delirious and demented patients are typically worse when they are alone or in unfamiliar surroundings, and at night. In functional psychiatric disturbances, symptoms tend to be more stable, or if they fluctuate, the fluctuation is related to specific stresses.

SECONDARY MANIFESTATIONS

The interaction of the primary disruption of brain function with the patient's psychology disturbs affect, behavior, perceptions, and personality to degrees that range from subtle to psychotic.

Affect. Emotional expression is appropriate to the content of thought but is labile and shallow, shifting rapidly but lacking real force. The patient may abruptly start laughing hysterically at a joke that is not that funny, only to burst into tears a minute later at a slightly sad thought. Delirious patients are more likely to be fearful, angry, or depressed, while demented patients are often depressed or apathetic.

Behavior. The general level of activity may be increased or decreased. Patients who are anxious are agitated, those who are depressed or apathetic are withdrawn, and those who are angry are belligerent or assaultive.

Perception. Illusions (misperceptions of actual stimuli) are the most common perceptual distortions. Hallucinations, which are sensory experiences in the absence of any external stimulus, may occur in any modality. Visual, olfactory, and tactile hallucinations occur more frequently in organic than in functional psychoses, but by itself no particular hallucination is diagnostic of an organic mental syndrome.

Personality change. Like anyone who must cope with a disturbing and unfamiliar situation, patients attempting to deal with the stress of an organic mental syndrome do more of what they ordinarily do to reduce anxiety and uncertainty. If they usually worry, for example, they may become obsessional. If they are belligerent when they are frightened, they may become assaultive when brain function is impaired. Habitually hypervigilant people may become paranoid, risk takers may become impulsive, and people who withdraw when they are upset may become uncommunicative when they develop an organic mental syndrome.

Psychosis. Psychotic symptoms (i.e., hallucinations, delusions, and gross impairment of reality testing) develop when an underlying psychosis such as schizophrenia is exacerbated by the stress of organic brain disease or when disturbances of memory, orientation, and perception disrupt the ability to distinguish internal from external reality. Delusions in organic mental syndromes usually concern everyday experiences; for example, fears of being harmed or attacked by medical staff who are mistaken for unknown tormenters. Organic delusions tend to be changeable and poorly organized. Hallucinations also vary from day to day and moment to moment. Some delirious patients experience intensely disruptive dream-like states (oneiroid states) in which they lose touch with reality and are flooded by hallucinations of frightening scenes, intense emotions, delusions, and violent impulses that may be remembered as actually having happened when the patient has recovered.

■ CATEGORIES OF ORGANIC MENTAL SYNDROMES

Depending on the primary and secondary disturbances that occur, organic mental syndromes are divided into several specific categories. Delirium, dementia, and some intoxication and withdrawal syndromes are associated with global disturbances, while signs and symptoms are limited to one area of functioning in the other disorders. When the etiology of an organic mental syndrome becomes clear (e.g., multi-infarct dementia, alcohol intoxication, or delirium due to hypoglycemia) the diagnosis is changed to organic mental disorder (e.g., organic mood syndrome caused by Cushing's disease is called organic mood disorder). Because these distinctions in terminology are primarily semantic, all organically induced changes in mood, behavior, thinking, and personality will be referred to collectively in this chapter as organic mental syndromes.

DELIRIUM

Delirium is an acute global disturbance of consciousness that is manifested by prominent disturbances of alertness, of the ability to shift and maintain the focus of attention, and of the level of awareness and activity. Symptoms may include disorientation, loss of short-term memory, clouded consciousness, confusion, disorganized thinking, perceptual disturbances, changes in psychomotor activity, and shifts in the sleep–wake cycle. Fluctuation is the hallmark of delirium. Not only do symptoms change dramatically and unpredictably, but the patient's overall state varies from obtunded to confused to apathetic to drowsy to restless to transiently alert.

DEMENTIA

Dementia is a chronic disturbance of memory, intellectual function, and judgment without prominent clouding of consciousness. Onset is generally more insidious than in delirium, and agitation is less prominent unless delirium is superimposed or the patient's surroundings are abruptly changed.

AMNESTIC SYNDROME

This syndrome consists of loss of short- and long-term memory in the absence of delirium or impairment of abstract thinking, judgment, and other higher cortical functions. Amnestic syndrome is caused by conditions that affect memory centers such as alcoholism and thiamine deficiency.

ORGANIC DELUSIONAL SYNDROME

In organic delusional syndrome, the major symptom is delusions induced by an organic factor in a patient who is not delirious. Temporal lobe epilepsy and drugs such as amphetamines, cocaine, bromocriptine, corticosteroids, propranolol, and indomethacin are the most common causes.

ORGANIC HALLUCINOSIS

In this disorder, hallucinations in the absence of delirium have an organic cause such as sensory deprivation, hallucinogens, stimulants, anticonvulsants, corticosteroids, digitalis, L-dopa, and ketamine.

ORGANIC MOOD SYNDROME

Manic or depressive symptoms not related to delirium have an organic etiology in this condition. Medications and illnesses that produce prominent mood changes without inducing alterations in consciousness or memory (Chapter 1) cause organic mood syndromes.

ORGANIC ANXIETY SYNDROME

Organic anxiety syndrome consists of panic or generalized anxiety caused by organic factors (Chapter 2) in the absence of delirium.

ORGANIC PERSONALITY SYNDROME

In organic personality syndrome, organic factors such as frontal lobe disease or temporal lobe epilepsy cause a personality disturbance or personality change involving mood swings, rage outbursts, poor judgment, apathy, or suspiciousness.

INTOXICATION AND WITHDRAWAL

Intoxications are substance-specific syndromes caused by ingestion of psychoactive substances. Withdrawals are specific syndromes caused by discontinuation or dosage reduction of these substances. Examples are considered in Chapter 6.

■ PRESENT ILLNESS

The possibility of an organic mental syndrome should be considered whenever a change in behavior, emotion, thinking, or personality develops in a patient who has an illness or is taking a medication or drug that could affect the brain. Organic mental syndromes are frequently to blame for acute changes in psychological status and for psychological syndromes that do not respond as expected to appropriate treatment. If psychiatric symptoms are severe, it may be easy to overlook the underlying physical condition.

■ PAST HISTORY

Many primary psychiatric syndromes, especially anxiety, depression, and schizophrenia, start relatively early in life, and are recurrent. Physical illness, on the other hand, becomes more frequent with age. Psychiatric symptoms that appear for the first time after early adulthood are therefore statistically more likely to be manifestations of an organic mental syndrome. A past psychiatric history does not exclude organic mental syndrome, however, since organic factors may coexist with or precipitate psychiatric disorders.

■ FAMILY HISTORY

If a patient has a family history that is consistent with the present symptoms (e.g., family history of depression, mania, or suicide in a patient who is now depressed), the case for a primary psychiatric diagnosis is strengthened. A family history of a neurological illness that can produce psychiatric symptoms, such as Huntington's or Wilson's disease, raises the suspicion of the same problem in the patient. Family histories are only suggestive, since genetic propensities to psychiatric disorders may be brought out by organic factors and primary psychiatric illnesses may develop in patients who do not have a positive family history.

■ ASSOCIATED PROBLEMS

Certain problems frequently complicate the management of organic mental syndromes, especially those noted below.

IMPULSIVITY

Conditions that affect the frontal lobes or that diffusely affect the brain reduce foresight and impair impulse control.

Suicidal and aggressive impulses are particular concerns because of fluctuating bursts of depressed or angry emotion, especially in delirious patients. It is therefore essential to observe patients with organic mental syndromes closely for destructive or self-destructive behavior that may erupt suddenly and unpredictably. The more acute the disorder and the more confused the patient, the greater the risk.

AGITATION

Patients who are frightened by their confusion frequently become agitated and combative. This problem is most likely to occur when the organic process worsens, when the patient is placed in unfamiliar surroundings, and at night (sundowning).

UNPREDICTABLE ASSAULTIVENESS

Some demented patients abruptly become violent without provocation, striking out, biting, spitting, or attacking others with no warning, after which they lapse back into their previous state.

SECONDARY DEPRESSION

Patients with chronic organic mental syndromes, especially dementia, often become depressed in reaction to helplessness, loss of function, and the primary effects of the organic disorder on brain systems that regulate emotion. Depression that occurs in the context of any irreversible illness is frequently more difficult to treat than primary depression.

■ LABORATORY FINDINGS

When they are positive, a few tests can be helpful in identifying organic mental syndromes, particularly delirium and dementia. Negative results do not exclude an organic mental syndrome.

ELECTROENCEPHALOGRAM (EEG)

The alpha rhythm on the EEG may be slowed in delirium (7). However, the slowing is relative to the patient's usual rhythm, and if this is toward the upper end of the normal range, the EEG in delirium may still be read as normal. Serial EEGs may demonstrate slowing when the patient's mental status is worse. Specific abnormalities are often, but not always, seen in epilepsy (less frequently when the lesion is subcortical), but the EEG usually is normal in dementia and in more focal organic mental syndromes such as organic mood syndrome.

AMYTAL INTERVIEW

Diffuse organic mental syndromes such as delirium and dementia are associated with depression of multiple brain functions. Drugs that further depress brain function such as barbiturates, benzodiazepines, and alcohol aggravate this disturbance and increase manifestations of the organic mental syndrome. The patient's reaction to the slow intravenous injection of a short-acting CNS depressant (e.g., 100–500 mg of amobarbital) therefore may be used to distinguish between odd or subtle syndromes in which it is not clear whether the etiology is functional or organic (8). If mental and behavioral symptoms increase, the disorder is more likely to be an organic mental syndrome. If symptoms resolve when the patient is sedated, a primary psychiatric etiology is more likely. Resuscitation equipment must be available in case the patient stops breathing. Barbiturates should not be administered to patients with porphyria, increased intracranial pressure, or allergy to the drug.

NEUROPSYCHOLOGICAL TESTING

Neuropsychological testing is a survey of cognitive, perceptual, intellectual, and motor function that can be helpful in distinguishing organic from functional mental syndromes (9). This all-day battery of tests also is used to document baseline functioning, follow deterioration and improvement, and suggest the level at which the patient can realistically be expected to function. Specialized training is necessary for psychologists to administer and interpret neuropsychological tests accurately.

TESTS FOR SPECIFIC SYNDROMES

Additional tests are dictated by specific signs and symptoms (6). For example, a computerized tomography (CT) scan should be considered in patients with focal signs, ataxia, or incontinence; lumbar puncture is indicated in patients with delirium and unexplained fever; and toxicology screening uncovers some but not all intoxications.

■ SUBTLE PRESENTATIONS OF DEMENTIA

A dementing illness may not be apparent for many years, especially in patients with initially superior intelligence and those who are socially adept enough to mask their deficiencies. Early manifestations of dementia in these patients are listed in Table 2 (10).

■ COURSE

The course of an organic mental syndrome depends primarily on the etiology. Delirium, which is usually caused by an acute

TABLE 2. **Early Signs of Dementia**

Depression
Irritability
Emotional outbursts
Uncharacteristic inability to get along with people
Accident proneness
Deteriorating job performance
Impulsivity
Indiscrete behavior
Poor judgment
Promiscuity
Personality change
Insomnia
Getting lost
Functional somatic complaints
Lateness
Feeling overwhelmed in new or complex situations
Repetitiousness
Inflexibility
Trouble balancing a checkbook
Perceptual illusions

insult, is reversible when the offending agent is treated or removed. However, because delirium is a sign of failure of an organ that is protected from many systemic influences, it may indicate that the underlying illness is severe and the long-term prognosis may be worse than if the patient had not become delirious. Dementia may be completely, partially, or not at all reversible. For example, dementia caused by pernicious anemia is completely curable, while Alzheimer's disease follows a progressive if unpredictable downhill course (6). No case of dementia should be assumed to be irreversible until aggressive attempts at treatment have consistently failed.

■ ETIOLOGY

Any physical factor that can directly or indirectly affect the brain can produce an organic mental syndrome. Emotional stress may predispose to delirium, but by themselves psychological factors never cause organic mental syndromes. Common etiologies of delirium and dementia are listed in Tables 3 and 4. Of these causes, medications and psychoactive substances are probably the most common. Causes of organic mood syndromes and organic anxiety syndromes are discussed in Chapters 1 and 2. Intoxication and withdrawal produced by psychoactive substances, which may produce delirium, dementia or more substance-specific syndromes, are addressed in Chapter 6.

TABLE 3. **Common Causes of Delirium**

Any prescription or nonprescription drug that affects the brain
Alcohol
Hypoxemia
Endocrine disorders (e.g., hypoglycemia, thyroid disease)
Organ failure in any system
Infections
Electrolyte disorders
Seizure disorders
Brain injuries
Metastatic cancer
Anemia

TABLE 4. **Common Causes of Dementia**

Any medication or drug, even in low doses
Alcoholism
Alzheimer's disease
Cerebrovascular disease (multi-infarct dementia)
Normal pressure hydrocephalus
Anemia
Nutritional deficiencies (e.g., B_{12}, folate)
Anemia
Posttraumatic states (e.g., after head injury, dementia pugilistica)
Chronic CNS infections (e.g., syphilis, fungal infections)
Hereditary and degenerative diseases (e.g., Huntington's disease,
    Creutzfeldt-Jakob disease, Wilson's disease)

■ DIFFERENTIAL DIAGNOSIS

Organic mental syndromes may mimic many other disorders (11, 12). Repeated testing may be necessary to uncover the primary disturbance.

MOOD DISORDERS

Impairment of concentration, attention, memory, and performance on neuropsychological testing associated with depression (depressive pseudodementia) may make it indistinguishable from dementia (see Chapter 1, Table 7). Both depression and mania can mimic the acute confusion, disorientation, and disorganization of delirium (pseudodelirium). The differential diagnosis is further complicated by the fact that delirium and dementia frequently are accompanied by dramatic emotional symptoms that may mistakenly be ascribed to important events in the patient's life. Mood disorders frequently coexist with organic mental syndromes, in which case the mood disorder may manifest itself as increased organic mental syndrome symptoms instead of an obvious change in emotional expression (i.e., aprosodia). A certain number of cases of depressive pseudodementia that remit initially with antidepressant therapy evolve months or years later into true dementia.

SCHIZOPHRENIA

Some clinicians equate any psychosis with schizophrenia. However, schizophrenia is much less common than delirium, organic delusional syndrome, and organic hallucinosis in a medical population. Any patient with an abrupt change in mental functioning should therefore be assumed to have an organic mental syndrome until proven otherwise (Table 5). Since schizophrenia may be precipitated by an organic mental syndrome, organic contributory factors should be considered even in clearly schizophrenic patients if they have deteriorated for no apparent reason.

SOMATIZATION

Functional somatic complaints are common in demented patients who are attempting to distract themselves from the primary disturbances of brain function. Features that distinguish these patients from those with somatoform disorders are discussed in Chapter 4.

TABLE 5. **Schizophrenia and Psychotic Organic Mental Syndromes**

Schizophrenia	Organic Mental Syndrome
Hallucinations most frequently auditory	Hallucinations in any modality; illusions common
Delusions complex, stable, complex, bizarre, and unlikely	Delusions concrete, changeable, and derived from real-life experiences
Gradual onset of psychosis	Abrupt onset in delirium; gradual in dementia
Symptoms begin in adolescence or early adulthood	Symptoms begin at any age
Psychosis recurrent or chronic; past history of psychosis common	Psychosis resolves with treatment of underlying illness; no past history unless previous OMS
Family history may be positive for schizophrenia	No psychiatric family history

DISSOCIATIVE DISORDERS

Dissociative disorders are functional alterations of consciousness, orientation, memory, feelings of reality, identity, or cohesiveness of the personality. In multiple personality disorder, two or more distinct personalities are capable of controlling a person's behavior. Psychogenic amnesia is an acute inability to remember significant information, and psychogenic fugue is an acute episode of travel away from home in which the patient forgets the past and assumes a new identity. Other dissociative disorders produce trance states, feelings of unreality or depersonalization, and various forms of automatic behavior. Differentiation of dissociative disorders from organic mental syndromes is summarized in Table 6.

PERSONALITY DISORDERS

Impulsivity and flagrant fluctuations of affect may mimic personality disorders that are characterized by flamboyant behavior and emotional instability. When maladaptive personality traits are exaggerated by organic mental syndromes, any personality disorder may be mimicked. Since personality disorders are evident by adolescence or early adulthood, an organic mental syndrome should be suspected whenever a personality change develops later in life.

■ TREATMENT

There are four phases in the treatment of organic mental syndromes: treatment of organic factors, behavioral management, involvement of the family, and use of medications (13, 14).

TREATMENT OF ORGANIC FACTORS

The first order of business in treating any organic mental syndrome is to identify and resolve organic factors that cause or contribute to the disorder.

1. Diagnose and treat reversible factors aggressively. Until the causative factor is removed, the organic mental syndrome is likely to continue.

TABLE 6. **Dissociative Disorders and Organic Mental Syndromes**

Dissociative Disorders	Organic Mental Syndrome
Memory loss limited to psychologically meaningful material	Loss of unimportant as well as meaningful memories
Long-term and short-term memory equally affected	Short-term memory more impaired than long-term memory
Disturbance of identity (i.e., disorientation to person) without disorientation to time and place	Disorientation to person only occurs if orientation to time and place are also lost
Acute symptoms improve temporarily with tranquilization	Tranquilizers exacerbate symptoms
Memory loss, confusion or personality change develop in context of emotional stress	Symptoms develop in the context of a physical illness or use of a medication or psychoactive substance
No fluctuation of symptoms except in reaction to stress	Symptoms fluctuate unpredictably
Past history of conversion or other psychogenic symptoms may be present	No past history of psychogenic physical or mental symptoms

2. Treat intercurrent conditions in dementia. Even minor metabolic imbalances, infections, or other disturbances can cause delirium in demented patients. It is therefore essential to ensure adequate hydration and nutrition, treat urinary and respiratory tract infections, and follow the patient's medical status closely.

3. Withdraw all unnecessary drugs. Virtually any medication can aggravate an organic mental syndrome. CNS depressants should be withdrawn gradually to avoid an abstinence syndrome.

4. Review the patient's use of prescription and nonprescription drugs and alcohol with the patient and the family. The patient may forget or conceal the number and variety of pills that

have been obtained from physicians, family members, and drug-
stores and may minimize the amount of alcohol that is being
consumed. Any one of these substances may contribute to an
organic mental syndrome.

BEHAVIORAL MANAGEMENT

The most common management problems in patients with
organic mental syndromes are agitation, emotional outbursts, and
noncompliance with treatments that the patient does not remember or cannot understand. These problems are addressed by com-
pensating for primary disturbances of memory, attention, orientation, and intellect.

1. Explain the problem. Most patients do not understand
that their confusion is due to the effects of a disease or medicine
on their brains. They become less frightened and agitated when
the cause of their symptoms is explained.

2. Be concrete and repetitive. The patient with a diffuse
organic mental syndrome such as delirium or dementia is not able
to think abstractly or to remember complex information. Any
explanations or instructions must therefore be simple and must be
repeated frequently. When the patient asks the same question
over and over it is a sign of forgetting, not manipulation. Important information should be repeated by the physician before the
patient has a chance to forget it.

3. Compensation for deficits in orientation and memory.
Agitation due to confusion and disorientation can be decreased by
reminding the patient of the location, why the patient is there,
and who the doctors and nurses are. A 24-hour clock, a calendar
on which the current date is indicated, and a night light help to
provide ongoing aids to orientation. If the patient is in the hospital, a room close to the nursing station facilitates frequent brief
visits by staff who can help to orient the patient.

*4. Minimize changes in environment, personnel, roommate,
and routine.* Patients with organic mental syndromes find it difficult to adapt to new or complex situations. If physicians, nurses,
other people, or the situation to which the patient has become
oriented change too frequently, the patient will not be able to
keep track of them and will become confused and agitated.

5. *Structure visits.* People the patient knows should be encouraged to be present around the clock to orient and reassure the patient. Visits by individuals the patient may find it difficult to remember should be limited or the patient may become more confused.

6. *Make use of remaining strengths.* Just because a patient is demented does not mean that important strengths do not remain. For example, an attorney might not be able to continue to practice law but might be able to function as an advisor to law students.

7. *Facilitate grieving.* Important functions that are lost as the result of a chronic organic mental syndrome must be mourned in the same way as any lost person or thing. Because the patient's intellectual capacities are limited, feelings about the loss must be discussed in simple terms and repeated frequently.

FAMILY INVOLVEMENT

The family can decrease confusion and agitation in hospitalized delirious or demented patients by providing familiar faces that are reassuring and orienting. When a patient with a chronic organic mental syndrome returns home, the family needs help in continuing to work with the patient (15).

1. *Be appropriately hopeful.* The family can usually be reassured that delirium is likely to resolve rapidly as the illness is treated. Even when a chronic organic mental syndrome cannot be cured, the family can expect that behavioral and emotional disturbances can be controlled and intercurrent conditions treated.

2. *Encourage grieving.* Just as the patient must grieve for lost function, the family must mourn the loss of the person they have known when a patient's cognitive or emotional functioning is permanently changed by a organic mental syndrome.

3. *Prevent burnout.* Families who expect themselves to care for a demented patient without any help or relief are liable to run out of emotional energy. Burnout can be minimized by encouraging them to take a vacation from the patient regularly, arrange for help in the home (e.g., from visiting nurses, homemakers, Meals on Wheels, and similar services), rotate responsibility among different family members, and express feelings of frustration and

helplessness openly. When the illness becomes too severe, or financial or emotional resources make it unrealistic to continue to care for the patient at home, the family should be helped to see that placement away from the home does not have to mean that they are completely abandoning the patient.

DRUG THERAPY OF ORGANIC MENTAL SYNDROMES

Medications are used in organic mental syndromes to treat anxiety, insomnia, depression, agitation, emotional outbursts, and memory loss (16–19).

1. Anxiety. Common causes of anxiety in patients with organic mental syndromes include confusion and disorientation, withdrawal from CNS depressants, and primary effects on the limbic system (e.g., in partial complex seizures). To treat these problems:

- Correct disorientation with behavioral approaches.
- Diagnose and treat abstinence syndromes (see Chapter 6).
- Treat seizure disorders with anticonvulsants.
- Use low doses of short-acting benzodiazepines (e.g., lorazepam, oxazepam), which are effective when given prn, and buspirone, which is not.
- Consider short-term administration of low doses of nonsedating neuroleptics but avoid long-term use whenever possible.
- Relaxation techniques and hypnosis usually are not helpful because the patient cannot concentrate well enough to use them.

2. Insomnia. Delirious patients often sleep during the day and are awake at night. Insomnia occurs in many patients with organic mental syndrome because they become disoriented and frightened when the lights are out. To treat insomnia:

- Keep a light on at night; have a person familiar to the patient in attendance if necessary.
- Use a low dose of a short-acting benzodiazepine (e.g., 0.125 mg

of triazolam) or an antihistamine (e.g., 25 mg of diphen-hydramine).

- If the patient is agitated at night, use a low dose neuroleptic (e.g., 0.5–2 mg of haloperidol or 10–25 mg of thioridazine).
- L-tryptophan plus vitamin B_6 is helpful to some patients.

3. Depression. A trial of an antidepressant frequently is indicated in dementia, even if a depressed mood is not apparent. When using an antidepressant in demented patients:

- Use nonsedating antidepressants with low anticholinergic potential such as desipramine or nortriptyline. Trazodone has been found to help a few demented, agitated patients.
- Begin with a low dose (e.g., 10 mg of desipramine) and increase the dose slowly (e.g., by 10 mg at a time).
- Consider a stimulant if the patient cannot tolerate a standard antidepressant.
- If the patient is severely depressed, consider ECT; dementia is not a contraindication.

4. Agitation and Assaultiveness. Delirious patients become combative when they are confused and disoriented. Demented and mentally retarded patients may become unpredictably assaultive. Possible drug treatments include:

- Oral nonsedating neuroleptics such as haloperidol, fluphen-azine, and thiothixene. Some clinicians prefer more sedating compounds such as thioridazine, but the anticholinergic and CNS depressant properties of these drugs may increase confusion. Whenever possible, low doses of a neuroleptic should be prescribed to coincide with anticipated episodes of agitation rather than on a regular basis. The risk of tardive dyskinesia is higher in patients with organic brain disease.
- Intravenous haloperidol and/or lorazepam (see Chapter 7). Severely agitated delirious and demented patients may be rapidly tranquilized with haloperidol alone, or in combination with lorazepam, without any further clouding of consciousness.
- Beta adrenergic blockers. Propranolol in a dose of 60–1000 mg per day titrated according to heart rate and clinical response diminishes unpredictable assaultive outbursts in brain dam-

aged patients. The drug must be given regularly, sometimes for as long as one month, to be fully effective. Severe bradycardia and hypotension are not common in demented patients taking high doses of propranolol if they are not very active physically.

- Antihistamines. Intramuscular or oral hydroxyzine can be used to sedate patients for an EEG, as it does not have a significant effect on the tracing.

  5. *Emotional outbursts and rage attacks.* Patients with personality disorders associated with low-grade brain damage may periodically become enraged or violent with minimal provocation. These patients sometimes benefit from:

- Carbamazepine, especially if EEG abnormalities are present
- Lithium, but confusion may be increased and neurotoxicity may be more likely than in patients with normal brain function
- Propranolol, as discussed above.

  6. *Memory loss.* Unless it is caused by depression, there is no proven treatment for organic memory loss. However, a number of experimental approaches have been tried, including:

- Lecithin may be given in a dose of 3–6 tablespoons per day.
- Physostigmine given intravenously may temporarily improve memory in Alzheimer's disease but is not a practical ongoing treatment.
- Ergot mesyloids (Hydergine) may improve depression and self-care somewhat in a dose of 6 mg/day for six months, but it probably does not benefit memory.
- Nimodipine is a centrally acting calcium channel blocker vasodilator that has been found helpful in preliminary trials in Europe.

■ REFERENCES

1. Lipowski ZJ: Transient cognitive disorders (delirium, acute confusional states) in the elderly. Am J Psychiatry 1983; 140:1426–1430
2. Folstein MF, Folstein SE, McHugh PR: "Mini-Mental State": a practical method for grading the cognitive state of patients for the clinician. J Psychiatr Res 1975; 12:189–198

3. Strub RL, Black FW: The Mental Status Examination in Neurology. Philadelphia, F.A. Davis, 1984

4. Jacobs JW, Bernhard MR, Delgado A, et al: Screening for organic mental syndromes in the medically ill. Ann Intern Med 1977; 86:40–45

5. Taylor MA, Sierles F, Abrams R: The neuropsychiatric evaluation, in Psychiatry Update: The American Psychiatric Association Annual Review, Volume 4. Edited by Hales RE, Frances AJ. Washington, DC, American Psychiatric Press, 1985

6. Benson DF, Blumer D (Eds): Psychiatric Aspects of Neurologic Disease, vol. 2. New York, Grune and Stratton, 1982

7. Engel GL, Romano J: Delirium: a syndrome of cerebral insufficiency. J Chronic Dis 1959; 9:260–266

8. Ward HG, Rowlett DB, Burke P: Sodium amylobarbitone in the differential diagnosis of confusion. Am J Psychiatry 1978; 135:75–78

9. Matarazzo JD, Matarazzo RG, Wiens AM, et al: Retest reliability of the Halstead Impairment Index in normals, schizophrenics and two samples of organic patients. J Clin Psychol 1976; 32:338–354

10. Wells CE: Dementia. Philadelphia, F.A. Davis, 1971

11. Lishman WA: Organic Psychiatry. New York, Blackwell, 1978

12. Wells CE: Pseudodementia. Am J Psychiatry 1979; 136:895–900

13. Hendrie HC (Ed): Brain disorders: clinical diagnosis and management. Psychiatr Clin North Am 1978; 1:1–193

14. Fauman MA: The emergency psychiatric evaluation of organic mental disorders. Psychiatr Clin North Am 1983; 6:233–257

15. Mace N, Rabins P: The Thirty-Six Hour Day. Baltimore, Johns Hopkins University Press, 1981

16. Adams F, Fernandez F, Anderson BE: Emergency pharmacotherapy of delirium in the critically ill cancer patient. Psychosomatics 1986; 27(suppl):33–37

17. Silver JM, Yudofsky S: Propranolol for aggression: literature review and clinical guidelines. International Drug Therapy Newsletter 1985; 20:9–12

18. Dubovsky SL, Ringel S: Psychopharmacologic treatment in neurology. Journal of Neurological Rehabilitation 1987; 1:51–66

19. Richelson E: Pharmacology of neuroleptics in use in the United States. J Clin Psychiatry 1985; 48:8–14

6 SUBSTANCE ABUSE AND DEPENDENCE

Pathological use of alcohol and psychoactive drugs (psychoactive substance use disorders) increasingly is being recognized as a major public health problem. The cost of substance abuse in lost productivity and in legal and medical expenses is over $100 billion per year (1). Alcoholism affects 10% of the population. Fifteen percent of American men and 9% of women have used narcotics other than heroin for nonmedical reasons. Between 1 and 3% of young adults have tried heroin and about one-fourth of young adults have used cocaine. During the first 18 months in which a cocaine hotline was established there were 450,000 callers, 90% of whom reported adverse consequences of cocaine abuse (2).

Substance use disorders are important problems in the medical setting for several reasons. Physical dependence occurs in at least 40% of patients taking recommended doses of benzodiazepines, and it is possible to become dependent on lower doses taken for long periods of time. In a general medical population, 20–50% of patients abuse one or more psychoactive substances (3). Medical and psychiatric complications of substance abuse and dependence are common, and problems with psychoactive substances complicate many medical and psychiatric disorders.

▪ DEFINITIONS

The terminology used to describe substance use disorders is continually being refined. *DSM-III-R* defines two categories related to psychoactive substances:

PSYCHOACTIVE SUBSTANCE DEPENDENCE

Psychoactive substance dependence is defined as at least three of a number of physical and behavioral problems related to continued substance use that have been present for at least one month or have been repeatedly present over longer periods of time, including:

1. use of the substance in larger amounts or for longer periods of time than the patient intended
2. unsuccessful attempts to control use of the substance
3. intoxication or withdrawal at work, at school, while taking care of children, when fulfilling other important roles, or when these syndromes are dangerous (e.g., while driving)
4. excessive amounts of time spent in obtaining or taking the substance or recovering from its effects
5. reduction in time spent in or abandonment of important activities because of use of the substance
6. continued use of the substance despite the knowledge that it is causing or exacerbating social, psychological, or physical problems
7. tolerance; i.e., decreased effect of the same amount of the substance, or increased amount of the substance, is necessary to produce the same effect
8. withdrawal symptoms when the substance is reduced in dose or discontinued
9. use of the substance to prevent or relieve withdrawal symptoms.

PSYCHOACTIVE SUBSTANCE ABUSE

Psychoactive substance abuse is defined as either of two symptoms of dependence lasting at least one month or recurring regularly over a longer time:

1. continued use despite knowledge that the substance is harmful
2. recurrent use of the substance in situations in which use is dangerous.

Many experts have expressed dissatisfaction with the imprecision of the term "addiction." Nevertheless, this term is still used in a number of settings to refer to severe dependence, overwhelming preoccupation with seeking and using psychoactive substances, and/or a high likelihood of relapse after the substance is successfully withdrawn.

■ SIGNS AND SYMPTOMS

In addition to the specific behaviors and physical symptoms that are used to define substance dependence and abuse, many patients with psychoactive substance use disorders have additional characteristics that need to be considered.

THINKING

Denial of the severity of the problem (or even that a problem exists) and the illusion of control over the substance are extremely common in people with substance use disorders. The beliefs that drug use is really not too serious or that it is just a symptom of other problems are particularly prevalent. Not infrequently, patients with escalating drug use claim that they can cut back whenever they choose; they have just not decided to do so.

BEHAVIOR

Patterns of pathological use of psychoactive substances may vary from daily use to excessive use only at certain times of the week (e.g., on weekends), to long periods of abstinence interspersed with binges lasting from days to months. Many patients use more than one substance, either sequentially or simultaneously.

SOCIAL FUNCTIONING

Many people begin using psychoactive substances believing that they function better when they are intoxicated. While it is true that small doses of CNS depressants or stimulants may transiently relieve anxiety or boredom or improve performance, long-term use inevitably impairs judgment, motor skills, and the ability to function as a worker, student, parent, spouse, and sexual partner. Patients who must use a drug to continue functioning— or at least to maintain the illusion of functioning—are already much more impaired than they believe. Continued use of substances such as cocaine, narcotics, and alcohol costs more and more in terms of energy, time, and money, bankrupting the patient socially, occupationally, and financially.

PHYSICAL STATUS

All psychoactive substances produce alterations in mood, thinking, behavior, and physiology when they are ingested (intoxication syndromes). Abstinence syndromes occur when the drug is abruptly withdrawn or significantly decreased in dose. There is a certain amount of overlap between the manifestations of intoxication and withdrawal from alcohol and other CNS depressants. The overall picture of intoxication and withdrawal syndromes with other psychoactive substances is more or less specific to each class of drug. Typical syndromes and their treatments are summarized in Tables 1, 2, and 3 (4–7).

■ CATEGORIES OF DEPENDENCE AND ABUSE

DSM-III-R classifies substance use disorders according to whether they involve each of 10 specific substances, multiple substances, or substances not included in the standard list such as anticholinergics and caffeine. Substances included in the nomenclature include alcohol, amphetamines or similarly acting sympathomimetics, cannabis, cocaine, hallucinogens, inhalants, opioids (narcotics), phencyclidine or similarly acting arylcyclohexylamines, sedatives, hypnotics or anxiolytics, and nicotine. All but one substance are said to produce dependence and abuse, while only dependence is diagnosed for nicotine.

■ PRESENT ILLNESS AND PAST HISTORY

Many patients progress to severe pathological use and more illicit drugs after a period of experimentation. For example, alcohol, tobacco, and marijuana frequently precede opioids in a patient's repertoire (8). While experimentation is not the same as regular use, positive experiences with one substance can encourage a person to increase the dose or move on to another drug (9). However, a group of middle class adults has recently become

TABLE 1. **Intoxication Syndromes**

Substance	Some Signs and Symptoms of Intoxication	Treatment
Alcohol	Overconfidence, impaired performance, mood swings, emotional outbursts, hyperactivity, hypothermia, tachycardia, dilated pupils, increased intracranial pressure, stupor, coma. Death rare with alcohol alone unless coma lasting more than 12 hours occurs.	Wait for alcohol to be metabolized Restrain Do not give tranquilizers or sedatives Haloperidol for agitation Keep warm Stimulants and caffeine do not hasten sobriety
Other CNS Depressants	Euphoria, increased seizure threshold, decreased pain threshold, sedation, paradoxical excitement, nystagmus, dysarthria, ataxia, postural hypotension, hypoxemia, hypothermia, respiratory depression, hyporeflexia, bullous skin lesions, necrosis of sweat glands. Short-acting drugs are more lethal.	Protect airway Oxygen and ventilation Keep warm I.V. fluids Maintain blood pressure with dopamine Alkalinize urine Dialysis if severe
Stimulants	Elevated mood, increased energy and alertness, decreased appetite, increased ability to perform boring tasks, hallucinations, manic behavior, fighting, hypervigilance, increased pulse and blood pressure, arrhythmias, seizures, delirium, paranoia	Neuroleptic for agitation and psychoses Phentolamine for increased pulse and blood pressure

Narcotics	Analgesia, drowsiness, euphoria, apathy, lethargy, itching, miosis, constipation, flushed and warm skin, hypotension, depressed reflexes, seizures, pulmonary edema, coma	Hydration Naloxone only for coma and apnea Protect airway
Hallucinogens and Cannabis Substances		
Hallucinogens	Dilated pupils, increased heart rate and blood pressure, hallucinations, illusions, depersonalizations, distorted sense of time, inappropriate affect, paranoia, anxiety	"Talking down" (reassurance in a quiet place) for "bad trips" Diazepam
Marijuana	Euphoria, anxiety and panic, increased appetite, tachycardia suggestibility, distortion of time and space, impaired motor skills, relapse in schizophrenia	"Talking down" (reassurance in a quiet place) for "bad trips"
Phencyclidine	As for hallucinogens, plus violence, psychosis, posturing, depression, bizarre behavior, mutism, echolalia, seizures, coma, analgesia, hypertension, nystagmus, ataxia, intracranial hemorrhage	Avoid any environmental stimulation I.V. haloperidol or diazepam for violence Restrain if necessary I.V. diazepam for seizures Avoid anticholinergic drugs
Anticholinergics	Confusion, delirium, hallucinations, amnesia, body image distortions, tachycardia, fever, warm and dry skin, dilated pupils, drowsiness, coma	Wait for drug to be metabolized I.V. physostigmine for coma or severe fever

TABLE 2. **Alcohol Withdrawal Syndromes**

Substance	Manifestations	Appears*	Lasts	Treatment
Alcohol withdrawal (shakes)	Coarse tremor of hands Nausea or vomiting Tachycardia, sweating, hypertension Anxiety, depression, or irritability Malaise or weakness Headache Insomnia	Hours	3 days–1 week	Thiamine and tapering dose of a benzodiazepine (e.g., chlorazepate, 60 mg on 1st day, 30 mg on 2nd day, 15 mg on 3rd day, then D/C.
Major motor seizures ("rum fits")	Major motor seizures in a small percentage of patients with the shakes	First 2 days	Briefly	No anticonvulsants unless patient is epileptic
Alcohol withdrawal delirium (delirium tremors or DTs)	Seizures precede other symptoms Delirium Autonomic hyperactivity (e.g., increased pulse rate, blood pressure, and sweating) Gross tremulousness Hallucinations	2–3 days	Up to 1 week	Hydration Thiamine Benzodiazepine (e.g., chlordiazepoxide, 200–400 mg/day) Neuroleptics for severe psychosis and agitation
Alcohol hallucinosis	Vivid auditory or visual hallucinations, usually threatening or derogatory in nature No command hallucinations	2 days	Hours–days; weeks–months in 10%; may become chronic	Neuroleptics if no spontaneous improvement

*Time after cessation of or significant decrease in drinking that syndrome begins.

directly involved with cocaine without using other substances first.

Patients may continue to drink or use drugs for some time before the extent to which use of the substance is controlling their lives becomes apparent. Denial by the patient, the family, and the patient's physician frequently contribute to this long prodromal period. The first indication of serious difficulty may be a social consequence, such as poor performance on the job or too much sick leave, or a medical complication such as abnormal liver function tests, an unexplained seizure, or a sudden psychosis. Erratic functioning in any important role should raise the index of suspicion for a substance use disorder. Every patient, regardless of the illness under consideration, should be asked in detail about use of alcohol and tobacco and about experience with other classes of legal and illegal psychoactive drugs.

■ FAMILY HISTORY

People whose parents or siblings use psychoactive substances are more likely to do so themselves. In the case of alcoholism, a genetic predisposition probably accounts for part of the increased risk (people with a family history of teetotalism are also more likely to become alcoholic, possibly because teetotalers avoid alcohol out of recognition of how easy it would be to become dependent). Family role modeling is a more important source of transmission of substance abuse and dependence for other drugs. Additional familial factors that increase the likelihood of problems with drugs and/or alcohol include family instability, parental rejection, divorce, and a chaotic or impoverished environment.

■ ASSOCIATED PROBLEMS

All psychoactive substances create costly and painful problems in the workplace. The accident rate on the job is increased three to four times in people with substance use disorders (7), and accident proneness in any setting is often an important clue to excessive use of drugs or alcohol. Marital and sexual dysfunction can also be produced by most substances. Additional problems may be associated with specific substances.

TABLE 3. **Abstinence Syndromes**

Substance	Manifestations	Appears*	Lasts	Treatment
Alcohol	See Table 2			
CNS depressants other than alcohol	Anxiety, irritability Orthostatic hypotension Autonomic hyperactivity Hyperreflexia Fever Diaphoresis Delirium Seizures Cardiovascular collapse	12–24 hours (7–10 days with long-acting benzodiazepines)	1 week (longer with long-acting drugs)	Barbiturate tolerance test followed by gradual withdrawal of phenobarbital
Stimulants	Depression, anxiety Irritability, anxiety	Hours–days	3–5 days	Imipramine for persistent depression

	Fatigue Increased or decreased sleep Nightmares Agitation Hyperphagia			Hospitalize for suicidal risk
Narcotics	Craving for drug Lacrimation and rhinorrhea Nausea and vomiting Restlessness and sleepiness Gooseflesh Dilated pupils Muscle aches Yawning Fever Insomnia Coryza	8–10 hours	7–10 days; subtle mood and sleep disturbances may persist weeks–months	Methadone 20–50 mg/day, decrease by 10–20%/day Clonidine 0.1–0.3 mg t.i.d. for two weeks

ALCOHOL

There are many physical complications of chronic alcohol use. Important examples include cerebral atrophy, Wernicke's encephalopathy, Korsakoff's syndrome, polyneuropathy, cardiomyopathy, myopathy, hypertension, gastritis, peptic ulcer, pancreatitis, cirrhosis, anemia, and impotence. Use of alcohol during pregnancy can cause the fetal alcohol syndrome in the fetus. This disastrous disorder is characterized by mental retardation, microcephaly, slowed growth, and facial anomalies.

SEDATIVES AND TRANQUILIZERS

Of those people who are not depressed when they begin using CNS depressants, up to 60% become depressed after 6 years of continuous use (10).

NARCOTICS

Between 50 and 87% of narcotic addicts have another psychiatric disorder, most commonly depression, anxiety, alcoholism, borderline personality, and antisocial personality (11). It may be difficult to determine whether these problems, particularly antisocial behavior, are primary or whether they result from effects of the drug or involvement with the drug culture. Crime is a common means of obtaining money for opioids and a major source of complications in narcotic users.

The death rate is increased 2–20 times in narcotic addicts. The unpredictable purity of street preparations makes fatal overdose an important contributing factor. Other sources of mortality include suicide, murder, anaphylactic reactions to intravenously injected impurities, and acquired immunodeficiency syndrome (AIDS) (up to two-thirds of patients in narcotic treatment centers are positive for HIV, and narcotic users die more rapidly of AIDS than other groups who acquire the virus[12]). Other infections are common, particularly venereal disease due to prostitution, hepatitis, endocarditis, septicemia, tetanus, and pulmonary, cerebral, and subcutaneous abscesses.

STIMULANTS AND CANNABIS

Chronic use of stimulants may be an attempt at self-treatment for attention deficit disorder, depression, and chronic dysphoria (unhappiness); more appropriate medications may reduce the need for the illicit drug. Cocaine may initially increase sexual desire, but with continued use it impairs sexual function. Rhinitis, sinusitis, and perforated nasal septum are common complications of intranasal use of cocaine, which also can cause hypertension, myocardial infarction, seizures, and sudden death (13). Infertility and passivity may be associated with chronic marijuana use.

■ LABORATORY FINDINGS

Blood and urine toxicology screening is now available for most psychoactive substances. Phencyclidine can be difficult to detect because it is recirculated in the enterohepatic circulation, similar to ethchlorvynol and glutethimide. Blood levels are zero in patients with abstinence syndromes. False positives and false negatives occur even with sophisticated testing.

Withdrawal from barbiturates and related compounds, benzodiazepines, and alcohol is diagnosed with the barbiturate tolerance test (Table 4), (14, 15). This test is performed by waiting until the patient shows definite abstinence signs or symptoms (e.g., tachycardia, hypertension, hyperreflexia, anxiety, tremulousness, or delirium) and administering 200 mg of pentobarbital or 60–100 mg of phenobarbital on an empty stomach. Patients who fall asleep are not tolerant and do not require further treatment. The amount of barbiturate needed to suppress withdrawal in all other patients is estimated from the response to pentobarbital or the amount of phenobarbital that produces intoxication. The patient is then stabilized for two to three days on that dose of barbiturate, and the drug is withdrawn gradually according to the protocol in Table 5. Phenobarbital is preferable to pentobarbital for the actual withdrawal because it is available in injectable form, and because its longer duration of action makes between dosage reemergence of the abstinence syndrome less likely. However, the drug may begin to accumulate after a few days, making more rapid dosage reduction necessary.

TABLE 4. Barbiturate Tolerance Test for Withdrawal from Barbiturates, Benzodiazepines, Alcohol, and Related Compounds

Pentobarbital Challenge (200 mg) *		
Response	**Degree of Tolerance**	**24-Hour Pentobarbital Requirement, mg**
Asleep	Minimal	None
Drowsy, ataxia, Mild dysarthria, nystagmus	Mild	400–600
Nystagmus only	Marked	600–1000
No response	Severe	1,000 + estimate from previous test

Phenobarbital Challenge *		
Give 60–100 mg phenobarbital every 2–6 hours until patient is intoxicated for 24-hour requirement.		

* Total daily barbiturate requirement calculated by either method is given in divided dose every six hours until patient stable for 2–3 days. Then reduce dose by 10% every 1–2 days. Treat re-emergence of withdrawal with slower dosage reduction and additional prn barbiturate. Withdraw more rapidly if patient becomes intoxicated.

30 mg phenobarbital = 100 mg pentobarbital

■ SUBTLE PRESENTATIONS OF SUBSTANCE DEPENDENCE AND ABUSE

Patients who are dependent on narcotics, tranquilizers, and sleeping pills may attempt to use the physician as a supplier. Behaviors listed in Table 5 raise the suspicion that a covert substance use disorder is behind visits to the physician.

■ COURSE

Exposure to "end stage" patients in medical school leads some clinicians to assume that substance dependence and abuse are inevitably chronic. In fact, two-thirds to three-fourths of patients respond to treatment. If they survive, the majority of nar-

TABLE 5. **Clues to Covert Substance Dependence**

Requests for a specific addicting drug

Lost prescriptions

Running out of medication before a prescription expires

Doctor shopping

Lying

Typical medical complications (e.g., elevated liver function tests)

Claim that a regular physician is unavailable to refill a prescription for a controlled drug

Threats, intrusiveness, or other attempts to coerce the doctor into writing prescriptions

Unexplained seizures, delirium, distress, or unusual behavior when access to substances is restricted (e.g., in the hospital)

Absence of intoxication in the presence of significant blood levels of a drug or alcohol

cotic addicts discontinue opioid use after about nine years. Relapse is common following successful therapy for any substance use disorder, however, so patient and physician must not interpret recidivism as a sign of failure or bad prognosis (16).

■ ETIOLOGY

People begin using psychoactive substances out of curiosity, because of peer pressure, or as a result of a wish to feel or function better or to be more relaxed. Initial experimentation usually occurs in a social setting, but later use is more solitary as the patient becomes increasingly isolated. Certain factors that cause or maintain pathological use of psychoactive substances deserve special attention (9, 17).

SELF-TREATMENT

Use of psychoactive substances to relieve depression, insomnia, anxiety, insecurity, mania, or hyperactivity creates a vicious circle that escalates drug use. If the substance does not aggravate the primary disorder, thereby making the patient want to take more of the drug, drug use continues or increases to prevent withdrawal.

ENCOURAGEMENT FROM THE SOCIAL SETTING

Pathological use of psychoactive substances is more likely in settings in which stress is high, drug use is condoned or encouraged, and drugs or alcohol are readily available. For example, more than 40% of enlisted men stationed in Vietnam—where heroin was easily available, cultural norms encouraged experimentation, and emotional pressure was extreme—reported trying narcotics at least once; one-half of these soldiers became dependent while in Vietnam. However, only a small number continued to use the drug after their return to the United States.

In this country, people who become dependent on narcotics tend to remain in the same peer group unless they are forcefully removed. In this case, they have a high risk of relapse when they return to the original situation. Narcotic use tends to be transmitted in epidemic fashion, with a dependent individual introducing the drug to friends and associates until everyone in a given social group has been exposed. Drug pushers are not an important source of new exposure, although they are clearly a major source for those who already are dependent.

REINFORCEMENT BY THE DRUG ITSELF

Most substances, especially opioids and stimulants, are potent reinforcers of their own use. This means that these drugs are so inherently rewarding that they make people want to take the drugs more. Patients who think that all they have to do to stop using psychoactive substances is to understand themselves better are ignoring the potent effect of the drugs in primarily increasing self-administration, regardless of the original motivation for drug use or the adverse consequences of continued dependence.

■ DIFFERENTIAL DIAGNOSIS

Differentiating between a primary psychiatric syndrome for which a patient uses psychoactive substances as a means of self-

TABLE 6. **Psychiatric Syndromes without an Organic Metal Syndrome That Can Be Mimicked by Substance Use or Withdrawal**

Substance	Syndromes
Alcohol	Depression Psychosis*
Stimulants	Paranoia Schizophrenia Mania
CNS depressants	Depression
Hallucinogens, PCP	Schizophrenia
Narcotics	Depression

* see Chapter 7

medication, and a primary substance use disorder that is causing secondary psychiatric symptoms, can be impossible while the patient is still using the substance. Most substance-induced syndromes (Table 1) resolve shortly after the substance is withdrawn, but stimulant-induced paranoia and psychosis, and alcohol-induced depression and hallucinosis, may persist for months. Common psychiatric disorders that can be mimicked by pathological substance use are listed in Table 6.

■ TREATMENT

Substance use disorders are treated in two phases. The goals of the initial phase are to withdraw the substance (detoxification), to help the patient recognize the problem, and to stabilize the environment. The second phase is directed toward longer-term management. Medications not involved in detoxification that may be helpful in both phases are discussed at the end of this section.

INITIAL TREATMENT

There is no point in engaging in long-term therapy before the patient is stabilized physiologically, psychologically, and socially. Steps taken during the early phase of treatment include (5, 9, 18):

DETOXIFY THE PATIENT

It is impossible to treat alcohol or drug use in patients who continue to use the substance. Patients who insist that they need to solve their emotional problems before they stop the substance need to be told that the substance is the problem, or at least part of it, and that other treatments cannot be instituted until drug use is discontinued. Reliable patients may be detoxified from tranquilizers, sedatives, and opioids by gradually reducing the dose (e.g., by 2–5 mg of diazepam every 1–4 weeks, more gradually for shorter acting benzodiazepines). Much of the time, however, detoxification involves substituting a medication listed in Tables 2 and 3 when signs of abstinence appear and gradually withdrawing the medication. Many compliant patients who abuse only one substance and who have strong psychosocial supports can be detoxified as outpatients. Outpatient detoxification is likely to fail when conditions listed in Table 7 are present. In these situations withdrawal should be conducted in a hospital or structured treatment center.

CONFRONT DENIAL GRADUALLY

One of the most significant obstacles to rehabilitation is the patient's denial of the problem. However, aggressive confrontation early in treatment may increase rather than overcome this defense. Denial is the patient's only means of dealing with guilt,

TABLE 7. **Indications for Inpatient Detoxification**

Failure of outpatient detoxification
Risk of dangerous abstinence syndromes
Coexisting medical or psychiatric illness requiring close observation
Insufficient psychosocial supports
Living situation encourages continued substance use
Readily available drugs at home
Lack of motivation
Strong denial
Severe impairment

shame, and anxiety, and stimulating these feelings before the patient has other means of coping with them only encourages abandoning the treatment to avoid the feelings, or encourages more drug use to control emotions that seemingly cannot be coped with in any other way. Patients who agree to detoxification without openly acknowledging the severity of substance abuse (usually to placate the family or the physician) do not have to be confronted immediately. As they feel more comfortable physically and gain some distance from the consequences of substance use, they are more likely to be able to begin to discuss ways in which the substance has affected their lives. Some patients need to suffer recurrent consequences of pathological substance use before they agree to detoxification and treatment. When continued denial leads to noncompliance and life- or health-threatening relapse, progressively stronger confrontation may be necessary.

CHANGE THE PATIENT'S ENVIRONMENT

Patients who return after detoxification to an environment in which drugs are readily available or in which the use of drugs or alcohol is condoned are likely to relapse rapidly. If this is a significant risk, the patient's living situation should be changed, for example, by transfer to a residential center or halfway house. After discharge, the patient may need to move or at least get a new phone number. All prescriptions written by other physicians should be discontinued, and alcohol should be removed from the home. The family should be enlisted to support the patient's abstinence and friends who use illicit drugs or drink heavily should be avoided, especially early in treatment, before the patient is able to resist their encouragement and modeling.

ONGOING TREATMENT

Substance use disorders are relapsing conditions that require an ongoing therapeutic commitment to the patient if therapy is to be successful. Principles of management during the postdetoxification phase include (11, 19, 20):

ESTABLISH A POSITIVE RELATIONSHIP

The patient must be seen regularly to monitor continued adjustment and use of drugs. In addition, the patient may need to substitute dependence on the physician and on other important people for dependence on the psychoactive substance.

ADOPT A DISEASE MODEL

Explaining chemical dependency as an illness helps the patient to stop seeing it as a moral failing that arouses guilt and shame, which are then suppressed with drugs and alcohol. The patient and the family should be educated about treatment principles, the risk of relapse, the self-perpetuating nature of substance use, and the manifestations and risks of intoxication and withdrawal.

TREAT ASSOCIATED PROBLEMS

When psychoactive substances are self-treatments for another psychiatric disorder, that disorder should be treated. However, unless psychiatric symptoms are extreme or clearly preceded substance use, it is usually reasonable to wait one to two months after detoxification to allow the effects of the substance on the brain to wear off before coexisting disorders are treated.

INSIST ON ABSTINENCE

If controlled use of addicting substances is possible in people who have been dependent on them, the few patients to whom this applies are too rare and difficult to identify to justify anything less than complete abstinence as a goal. A trial period of abstinence, say for a month or even for a few weeks, may help the patient to feel so much better that continued abstinence becomes easier. The patient should avoid *all* potentially habituating substances, not just the one on which dependence occured.

ASSESS MOTIVATION

The most concrete sign of the patient's motivation to improve is willingness to abstain from all drugs and alcohol. Patients who insist that they can control use of psychoactive substances or who demand another drug that causes dependency have not yet made a commitment to address their problem seriously. These patients need continued discussion of their denial of their inability to control the use of the substance.

INVOLVE THE FAMILY

Family members and friends often are aware of relapses that are concealed by the patient. They may also be a source of prescription or nonprescription drugs, they may otherwise encourage use of the substance, or they may require treatment for dependency themselves. A spouse may be successful in coercing into treatment a patient with a severe substance use disorder who adamantly refuses help by threatening to leave the patient if the situation does not change. Such threats should never be employed unless the spouse is truly committed to acting on them.

ARRANGE PERIODIC TOXICOLOGY SCREENS

Unscheduled urine screens can be essential in identifying relapse and noncompliance before the problem becomes as blatant as it was prior to treatment, and in enforcing contingency contracts (described below). The risk of cheating on the urine sample is minimized if the patient is required to produce it under observation.

AVOID MEDICATIONS THAT CAN CAUSE DEPENDENCE

Unless they are clearly indicated for acute pain or time-limited acute anxiety, opioids, antianxiety drugs, and hypnotics should not be prescribed for patients who have used any psychoactive substance excessively in the past.

HELP THE PATIENT TO RECOGNIZE EMOTIONS AND SITUATIONS THAT LEAD TO SUBSTANCE ABUSE

Many patients do not realize that they use psychoactive substances when they are upset or under stress because the situations in which the drug is used have become associated in their minds with intoxication rather than distress. Reviewing in detail exactly when the patient uses drugs or alcohol can identify situations and emotions that the patient must learn to handle in other ways.

ENCOURAGE EXERCISE

Exercise lasting more than 20 minutes at a time may reduce drug craving through release of endorphins.

REFER TO SELF-HELP GROUPS

Peer support groups now exist for people who have had problems with alcohol (Alcoholics Anonymous), narcotics (Narcotics Anonymous), cocaine (Cocaine Anonymous), and multiple substances (Drugs Anonymous). These groups offer encouragement from people who have had similar experiences, emotional sustenance, and confrontation that may be more credible than interventions by professionals. Most self-help groups are listed in the local telephone directory.

RECOMMEND RESIDENTIAL TREATMENT FOR UNRELENTING OR FREQUENTLY RELAPSING SUBSTANCE USE DISORDERS

When the environment encourages continued use of psychoactive substances and supports are weak or ineffectual, therapeutic communities and other residential programs may be necessary. These nonhospital programs provide a structured setting, powerful peer input, a drug-free environment, and professional supervision until the patient is better able to resist pressures for substance use or until the patient is able to move to a different location.

CONSIDER SANCTIONED TREATMENT AND CONTINGENCY CONTRACTING

Patients who are forced to remain in treatment do better than those who are free to terminate therapy as soon as they feel uncomfortable. Legally sanctioned treatment—for example, making retention of a driver's license or suspension of a jail sentence for drunken driving contingent on successful completion of an alcoholism program—is one way to accomplish this goal. In contingency contracting, the patient agrees in advance to some negative consequence in the event of a positive urine screen, failure to obtain a scheduled urine test, or withdrawing from therapy. One popular negative contingency is a letter written by the patient and held by the physician that reveals the substance use disorder to an employer or licensing body and requests suspension of employment or of a professional license. The letter is mailed immediately if the patient lapses. The contingency may also be positive. For example, the patient or the family may leave a sum of money with the physician at the beginning of treatment.

The patient is then paid back a certain amount for every week of sobriety, clean urine, or success in therapy.

EXPECT RELAPSES

Return to substance use does not indicate that the treatment will not eventually be successful. Relapses should be dealt with in a nonjudgmental manner, and detoxification and hospitalization should be arranged rapidly if they become necessary.

LEAVE THE DOOR OPEN

Some patients who have persistently refused treatment eventually agree to therapy when they have experienced a sufficient number of adverse consequences. They should be invited to enter treatment with each rehospitalization or complication.

DRUG THERAPY OF SPECIFIC SUBSTANCE USE DISORDERS

Certain medications are used routinely or experimentally in the treatment of alcohol, narcotics, and cocaine dependence.

ALCOHOLISM

The pharmacologic cornerstone of alcoholism treatment is disulfiram (Antabuse). This drug interacts with alcohol to produce nausea, vomiting, discomfort, headache, diaphoresis, headache, flushing, difficulty breathing, and hypertension. Anticipation of the alcohol–antabuse reaction helps the patient to avoid impulsive drinking, although the binge drinker may discontinue the medication a few days before an anticipated bout of drinking. The reasons would have to be compelling not to prescribe disulfiram for alcoholics who have difficulty remaining abstinent. The initial dose is 500 mg at bedtime for a week, followed by 250 mg at bedtime. Major side effects include rash, GI distress, and acne. Disulfiram may increase blood levels of oral anticoagulants and phenytoin. The only real contraindication is organic brain disease severe enough to interfere with the patient's understanding of the use of the drug.

NARCOTICS

Three medications have been used as adjuncts in the management of individuals who have been dependent on narcotics:

1. Methadone is used to withdraw narcotics during detoxification. During maintenance therapy it is used to decrease craving for opioids and maintain patients in close contact with narcotic treatment centers, where they must go every day to obtain the medication. Detoxification using methadone is summarized in Table 3. The usual maintenance dose is 40–80 mg/day. When the patient is stable, reduction of the dose by 1 mg/week or less may be attempted. Abstinence symptoms are common when the dose of methadone is reduced below 20 mg per day in narcotics addicts. Any physician may use methadone to treat acute or chronic pain, even in a narcotic dependent patient, but methadone maintenance for addiction can only be carried out in a federally approved program with patients with clearcut signs of dependence.

2. L-alpha-acetylmethadol (LAAM) is a long-acting synthetic narcotic substitute that has been used experimentally in the same way as methadone. Because it suppresses withdrawal for 72 hours, it is necessary to administer LAAM only three times per week. However, more patients drop out of narcotic treatment programs using LAAM than those using methadone.

3. Naltrexone is a narcotic antagonist used in a manner analagous to disulfiram. A dose of 100–150 mg of naltrexone three times per week precipitates an abstinence syndrome when a patient uses a narcotic. The attrition rate is very high in patients using this drug.

COCAINE

There is no specific antagonist or maintenance drug that can substitute for cocaine. However, in preliminary studies, imipramine and desipramine have been shown to decrease craving for cocaine, attenuate cocaine-induced euphoria, and reduce the risk of relapse, even if the patient is not depressed to begin with. Lithium may also attenuate euphoria induced by cocaine and stimulants, but it does not appear to be as effective as imipramine and desipramine. Amantadine may decrease craving for cocaine, but it has not been tested in double-blind studies.

■ ADDICTED PHYSICIANS

Physicians, nurses, and other health care professionals have higher rates of dependency on narcotics than other professionals of comparable education and socioeconomic status. Yet until recently, the importance of substance use disorders in this group was underrecognized. As a result, many affected health care personnel did not receive adequate treatment.

Physicians initially begin using narcotics to relieve physical discomfort, anxiety, depression, fatigue, or the stresses of their work rather than to experience euphoria. However, once they become dependent on a drug or alcohol their pattern of use and impairment are the same as any other individual with a substance use disorder. The only meaningful differences are that the incidence of personality disorders is probably less in physicians who are dependent on narcotics than it is in other narcotic users, and that physicians find it easier to obtain drugs of dependency at work.

With appropriate treatment, the rate of cure of substance use disorders in physicians is as high as 80%. This high rate of success depends on a two-pronged approach in addition to standard treatments:

PEER REPORTING

It is only too common that colleagues know about a physician's dependence on drugs or alcohol. Even though the physician may be severely impaired, denial, identification with the physician, reluctance to seem like an informer, and unwillingness to face an unpleasant confrontation all play a role in not insisting that the physician seek help. To combat the tendency of doctors to avoid dealing with use of psychoactive substances by their colleagues, many states now require that any physician with knowledge that is not obtained in the context of a doctor–patient relationship of another doctor's dependence report the problem to an agency connected with the licensing body. The agency offers a confidential evaluation, over the physician's objections if necessary. No action is taken if the report is unfounded. However, if a problem exists, the physician is required to seek treatment or be reported to the licensing board.

If physician impairment is to be prevented during practice, alertness to problems with psychoactive substances in one's colleagues must begin in medical school. Anyone who suspects such a problem should attempt to discuss it with the student or the physician involved, urging him or her to seek help. If a colleague with a substance use disorder refuses to be treated, or if it is too uncomfortable to discuss the situation with the person involved, it is essential to consult with one of the student or physician assistance programs affiliated with medical schools and local medical boards.

CONTINGENCY CONTRACTING

As is true in other settings, treatment of drug and alcohol dependence in physicians is most likely to be successful when the physician is coerced into completing treatment. In contingency contracting for physicians, the most powerful negative contingency is surrender of the medical license. Treatment carried out with the threat that the physician will not be able to practice if treatment is not successful is very likely to be effective.

■ REFERENCES

1. Research Triangle Institute: The Study of the Economic Costs to Society of Alcohol, Drugs and Mental Disorders. Research Triangle Institute, Research Triangle Park, NC, 1981
2. Kozel NJ, Adams EH (Eds): Cocaine Use in America: Epidemiologic and Clinical Perspectives. NIDA Research Monograph Series no. 61. Rockville, MD, National Institute on Drug Abuse, 1985
3. Crowley TJ, Chesluck D, Pitts S, et al: Drug and alcohol abuse among psychiatric admissions: a multidrug clinical toxicologic study. Arch Gen Psychiatry 1974; 30:13–20
4. Pearlson GD: Psychiatric and medical syndromes associated with PCP abuse. Johns Hopkins Medical Journal 1981; 148:25–33
5. Khatzian EJ, McKenna GJ: Acute toxic and withdrawal reactions associated with drug use and abuse. Ann Intern Med 1979; 90:361–372
6. Thompson WL: Diazepam and paraldehyde for treatment of severe delirium tremens. Ann Intern Med 1975; 82:175–180
7. Ellinwood EH, Woody G, Krishnan RR: Treatment for drug abuse, in Psychiatry. Edited by Michels R, Cavenar JO, Brodie HKH, et al. Philadelphia, J.B. Lippincott, 1986

8. Kandel D, Single E, Kessler RC: The epidemiology of drug use among New York state high school students. Am J Public Health 1976; 66:45–53

9. Millman RB: General principles of diagnosis and treatment, in Psychiatry Update: The American Psychiatric Association Annual Review, vol. 5. Edited by Frances AJ, Hales RE. Washington, DC, American Psychiatric Press, 1986

10. O'Brien CP, Woody GE: Sedative-hypnotics and antianxiety agents, in Psychiatry Update: The American Psychiatric Association Annual Review, vol. 5. Edited by Frances AJ, Hales RE. Washington, DC, American Psychiatric Press, 1986.

11. Jaffe JH: Opioids, in Psychiatry Update: The American Psychiatric Association Annual Review, vol. 5. Edited by Frances AJ, Hales RE. Washington, DC, American Psychiatric Press, 1986

12. Rothenberg R, Woelfel M, Stoneburner R, et al: Survival with the acquired immunodeficiency syndrome: experience with 5,833 cases in New York City. N Engl J Med 1987; 317:1297–1302

13. Taylor D, Ho BT: Neurochemical effects of cocaine following acute and repeated injection. J Neurosci Res 1977; 3:95–101

14. Smith DE, Wesson DR: Phenobarbital technique for treatment of barbiturate dependence. Arch Gen Psychiatry 1971; 24:56–60

15. Wikler A: Diagnosis and treatment of drug dependence of the barbiturate type. Am J Psychiatry 1968; 125:758–765

16. Simpson DD, Joe GW, Bracy SA: Six-year follow-up of opioid addicts after admission to treatment. Arch Gen Psychiatry 1982; 39:1318–1326

17. Robbins LN, Helzer JE, Davis DH: Narcotic use in Southeast Asia and afterwards. Arch Gen Psychiatry 1975; 32:955–961

18. Charney DS, Steinberg DE, Kleber HD: The clinical use of clonidine in abrupt withdrawal from methadone. Arch Gen Psychiatry 1981; 381:273–277

19. Kissen B, Begleiter H (Eds): The Biology of Alcoholism. New York, Plenum, 1977

20. Rose A: Psychotherapy and Alcoholics Anonymous: can they be coordinated? Bull Menninger Clin 1981; 18:229–249

7 PSYCHOSIS

Psychoses not caused by organic mental syndromes (i.e., functional psychoses) are relatively rare in nonpsychiatric practice. For example, schizophrenia occurs in less than 1% of the population, although one-half of the mental hospital beds in this country are occupied by schizophrenics. However, even the student who does not plan to enter psychiatry must know how to manage agitation and disorganization caused by acute psychoses. Patients with recurrent or chronic psychoses occupy an inordinate amount of any physician's time, utilizing more health care services than nonpsychiatric patients, while frequently exhibiting noncompliance and unpredictability in working with the physician.

■ SIGNS AND SYMPTOMS

Psychosis is present when reality testing is grossly impaired. Typical manifestations include delusions, hallucinations, inability to communicate, and severely disorganized, suspicious, withdrawn, or exalted behavior.

DELUSIONS

Delusions are fixed, false ideas that are inconsistent with a patient's culture or religion and cannot be corrected by rational arguments. Delusions may be poorly organized and changeable, as in organic mental syndromes, or complex and systematized, as in many functional psychoses. Delusions that bear an identifiable relationship to a depressed or elated mood (e.g., delusions of being punished, of having sinned, or of being immensely powerful) are said to be mood-congruent; delusions that are not obviously related to a change in mood are mood-incongruent.

HALLUCINATIONS

Hallucinations are perceptual experiences that occur in the absence of an actual stimulus. Any psychosis may be associated with hallucinations in any sensory modality, but olfactory, tactile, and complex visual hallucinations are more common in psychotic organic mental syndromes.

DISTURBANCES OF SPEECH AND THOUGHT

Psychotic speech may be incoherent, fragmented, or incomprehensible. Loose associations, which are seen most commonly in schizophrenia, are connections between ideas that have a personal, idiosyncratic meaning that makes it difficult or impossible to follow the patient's logic. Dysphasias and paraphasias (incorrect, often nonsensical substitutes for a particular word that resemble that word in some way) are typical of organic brain disease, but they may be difficult to distinguish from schizophrenic neologisms, which are words invented by the patient out of some private meaning. Circumstantial speech follows a roundabout path but eventually returns to the point, while tangential speech digresses to a new idea before the first idea is completed. Flight of ideas, which is characteristic of mania, is an extreme form of tangentiality in which logical connections may be missed because they go by so rapidly. By itself, no disorder of speech is pathognomonic of any particular psychosis.

Virtually all psychoses exhibit disturbances in the content of thought (e.g., abnormal thoughts such as delusions). Some clinicians believe that schizophrenia is more likely than other psychoses to be associated with a formal thought disorder (i.e., a disorder of the form of thinking) in addition to disturbed thought content. Other experts find that a formal thought disorder is equally likely to be present in schizophrenia, mania, or depression. A formal thought disorder has the following characteristics:

Loose associations. These may be demonstrated by asking the patient to give the most general meaning of common sayings or similarities among different objects. Examples of loose associations are interpreting the proverb "a rolling stone gathers no moss" as "to move is to perish"; and saying that a table and a chair are alike because "they sit together to pray."

Concrete thinking. Inability to abstract beyond the immediate meaning of an idea (e.g., the meaning of "a rolling stone gathers no moss" is "because it keeps moving"; or "a hammer is like a screwdriver" because "they go together") is characteristic of schizophrenia, delirium, and dementia.

Thought blocking. Blocking is sudden cessation of the patient's train of thought, after which it takes off in an entirely different direction. People who are very distracted may appear to have this problem.

Idiosyncratic logic. The schizophrenic patient often uses peculiar forms of logic. An example is syllogistic thinking, in which the patient reasons, "chimpanzees have two arms and two legs; I have two arms and two legs; therefore, I am a chimpanzee."

Other abnormalities of the form of thought. These may include echolalia (rote repetition of others' words), circumstantiality, perseveration, tangentiality, and derailment, among others.

BEHAVIORAL DISTURBANCES

The majority of psychotic patients are unable to function at their usual or even a barely acceptable social or occupational level. They may be severely withdrawn or greatly excited and agitated. The manic patient frequently is intrusive; psychotically depressed patients tend to be emotionally inaccessible; and schizophrenic patients are more likely to be grossly inappropriate, bizarre, withdrawn, unexpressive, or inept. The behavior of patients with psychotic organic mental syndromes is characterized by unpredictable fluctuation, often between agitated and confused assaultiveness and stuporous withdrawal.

POSITIVE AND NEGATIVE SYMPTOMS

Some clinicians classify symptoms of schizophrenia according to whether they are positive or negative. Positive symptoms are defined by the presence of some positive abnormality such as agitation, hallucinations, or delusions. Negative symptoms refer to the absence of some important characteristic. Examples include social withdrawal, poverty of speech, lack of motivation, difficulty paying attention, low energy, apathy, and blunting of emotional expression (1). Positive symptoms are more likely than negative symptoms to respond to most of the drug therapies currently available in the United States.

■ CATEGORIES OF PSYCHOSIS

If they are severe enough, mania and depression may be associated with psychotic symptoms that usually are consistent with their mood (see Chapter 1). The other major psychotic disorders are described in the following sections.

SCHIZOPHRENIA

Schizophrenia is a chronic mental disorder that must be continuously present for at least six months, including at least one week of active psychosis (less if the patient is rapidly treated), in order to be diagnosed according to current criteria. The disorder consists of active, prodromal, and residual symptoms that alone or in combination lead to deterioration of such functions as work, interpersonal relationships or self-care, or to failure to achieve expected level of development in childhood or adolescent schizophrenics. Symptoms of schizophrenia may vary during different phases of the illness.

The *prodromal phase* precedes active psychosis. Prodromal symptoms are attenuated versions of more blatant psychotic symptoms. Typical examples are listed in Table 1. The same

TABLE 1. **Prodromal and Residual Symptoms of Schizophrenia**

Social isolation or withdrawal

Marked impairment of functioning in social, occupational, or student role

Impaired personal hygiene and grooming

Blunted or inappropriate affect

Marked lack of initiative, interest, or energy

Bizarre behavior (e.g., talking to self in public or collecting garbage)

Peculiar beliefs or magical thinking inconsistent with cultural norms (e.g., beliefs in clairvoyance or telepathy or feelings that others are talking about the patient in secret)

Unusual perceptual experiences (e.g., recurrent illusions or sensing the presence of a mysterious force)

symptoms are observed during the *residual phase*, which follows a period of active psychosis.

The *active phase* is characterized by such symptoms of clearcut psychosis as:

- *delusions* that are bizarre or implausible: for example, that others can hear the patient's thoughts; that the patient is being controlled by an outside force; or that thoughts are being inserted into or withdrawn from the patient's mind
- *hallucinations:* for example, of voices commenting on the patient's behavior or thoughts, or of two or more voices talking to each other
- *incoherence* or marked *loosening of associations*
- *catatonia*, consisting of gross purposeless excitement and agitation, or withdrawal and mutism, rigidity, negativistic resistance to all instructions or attempts to move the patient, or bizarre posturing
- *flat or inappropriate affect* (emotional expression that is a monotone or is grossly inconsistent with the content of thought)

If delusions or hallucinations are mood-incongruent, these alone are sufficient to diagnose the active phase of schizophrenia. If they are mood-congruent, at least one other symptom must be present to warrant the diagnosis.

Schizophrenia currently is divided into five subtypes. The *catatonic* type is characterized by prominent catatonia in addition to typical schizophrenic symptoms. The *disorganized* type is dominated by incoherence, marked loosening of associations, grossly disorganized behavior, and flat or inappropriate affect. In the *paranoid* type, there are one or more systematized delusions or auditory hallucinations related to a single theme. The *undifferentiated* type is a subcategory in which psychotic symptoms do not meet specific criteria for another subtype, while patients with the *residual* type exhibit residual but not active symptoms (refer to Table 1).

SCHIZOPHRENIFORM DISORDER

DSM-III-R defines schizophrenia as a disorder that is continuously present for at least six months. Psychoses in which typical acute, prodromal, and/or residual symptoms of schizophrenia have been present for less than six months are labeled schizophreniform in order to preserve the concept of schizophrenia as a chronic condition. Some patients with schizophreniform disorder may have a disorder that is distinctly different from schizophrenia and that may be more closely related to mania or depression. Patients with schizophreniform disorder who remain continuously impaired for more than six months are rediagnosed at that time as schizophrenic.

SCHIZOAFFECTIVE DISORDER

A few patients exhibit mixtures of schizophrenic and mood symptoms in which neither one clearly causes the other. For example, the patient may have been depressed or elated but continues to have delusions and hallucinations after mood has become stable; or the patient may have both depression and loose associations. There is disagreement about whether this is a distinct disorder, a combination of schizophrenia and a mood disorder, or an unusual variant of one or the other condition.

BRIEF REACTIVE PSYCHOSIS

Brief reactive psychosis is an acute psychotic condition lasting less than one month, in which symptoms that appear schizophrenic develop during a time of significant stress. Psychosis is accompanied by confusion or by rapid shifts from one emotion to another. The patient has no prodromal symptoms of schizophrenia, does not have a life-long history of withdrawn or eccentric behavior, and recovers completely from the psychosis. Patients with personality disorders (especially borderline personality) are prone to develop brief reactive psychoses in the context of substance abuse, loss, or an intense relationship, especially with a psychotherapist or physician. No matter how schizophrenic these patients may seem acutely, they have a different disorder that requires a different treatment strategy.

DELUSIONAL DISORDER (PARANOIA)

In delusional disorder, the patient is preoccupied by delusions involving situations that could conceivably occur in real life such as being followed, poisoned, sick, in danger, or loved at a distance. Hallucinations and typical schizophrenic, manic, or depressive symptoms are not prominent. The patient may make elaborate plans based on the delusions (e.g., complaining to the police, visiting physicians, or attacking the presumed persecutor), but behavior is not otherwise disorganized and it may be possible to function in a structured social or occupational role. Six subtypes of delusional disorder have been defined, depending on the predominant type of delusion: *erotomanic* type (delusion that a person of higher status is in love with the patient); *grandiose* type (delusions of inflated power, self-worth, knowledge, identity, or special relationship to a grandiose figure); *jealous* type (delusion that a sexual partner is unfaithful); *persecutory* type (delusion that the patient or someone close to the patient is being persecuted or is in danger); *somatic* type (delusion of having a physical defect, disease, or disorder); and *unspecified* type (mixed or atypical delusions).

ATYPICAL PSYCHOSIS (PSYCHOTIC DISORDER NOT OTHERWISE SPECIFIED)

This is a category for psychoses that do not meet formal criteria for other psychotic disorders. There are a number of unusual syndromes that do not seem to be caused by organic mental syndromes that are called atypical; for example, delusions that a benign force is watching over the patient, or persistent auditory hallucinations with no other symptoms. A few odd psychoses are encountered only in certain cultures; for example, the delusion seen in some dwellers in the northwoods that the patient has become a flesh-eating monster (whitigo or wendigo). Only further research will determine whether these are distinct psychoses or variants of better established diagnostic categories. It also is possible that the currently accepted categories will be further subdivided when more knowledge is gained about subtle variations in their manifestations.

■ HISTORY

A careful history is frequently the only way to distinguish among different psychotic disorders. Facets of the present illness, past history, and family history that deserve special attention are summarized in Table 2.

■ ASSOCIATED PROBLEMS

Clinicians in any setting may have to contend with the more significant complications of psychosis:

SUBSTANCE ABUSE

It is not uncommon for patients to abuse nonprescription drugs and alcohol in an attempt to control chronic psychotic symptoms. When the substance is withdrawn, psychotic symptoms that reemerge may be mistaken for an abstinence syndrome. Some younger psychotic patients purposely use drugs such as stimulants and hallucinogens that aggravate the symptoms from which they suffer in the first place. At the cost of becoming more disorganized, they feel a sense of control over phenomena that they are producing themselves instead of experiencing helplessly.

ASSAULTIVENESS

The majority of psychotic patients are not dangerous. Occasionally, however, delusional ideas of being persecuted or of having special powers may make patients with paranoid disorder or schizophrenia assaultive, and some manic patients may become violent if their unrealistic plans are interrupted. Rarely, psychotically depressed patients kill family members and then themselves out of a delusional belief that they would be too miserable if they went on living. Any acutely psychotic patient who feels threatened and disorganized may become belligerent if the environment does not feel safe. Impulse control in psychoses usually improves with treatment of the underlying disorder.

HOMELESSNESS

With deinstitutionalization of the chronic mentally ill, some patients who were relatively well adjusted to the structured routine of a mental hospital were deemed not to be disturbed enough to require further inpatient treatment. It was hoped that these

TABLE 2. **Common Historical Findings in Selected Psychotic Disorders**

Aspect of History	Schizophrenia	Mood Disorder	Organic Mental Syndromes	Brief Reactive Psychosis
Age of onset	15–35, usually late teens to mid-20s	Early 20s (bipolar) to later life (unipolar) Psychotic depression	Any age	Usually 20s and 30s
Mode of onset	Insidious; psychosis may develop over months or years	Rapid (mania) to gradual (depression)	Abrupt	Rapid to abrupt
Premorbid functioning	Socially isolated; eccentric; detached; defective emotional rapport;	Overinvolved and hyperactive, possibly successful (mania) or pessimistic, hard-	None unless pre-existing mental illness is present	Unstable relationships; intense, changeable emotions;

	cognitive disturbances	working and sensitive to loss (depression)		manipulative suicide attempts; substance abuse; unsuccessful psychotherapy
Course	Chronic; deteriorating functioning	Exacerbations and remissions, with return to premorbid or, at least, effective level of functioning	Remits completely when underlying illness treated. Increased risk of physical morbidity subsequently	Remits rapidly with structure
Psychiatric family history	Schizophrenia	Depression, mania, suicide, alcoholism, antisocial behavior	None	Mood disorder; personality disorder

individuals could receive outpatient care in the neighborhood mental health center system and local clinics, and in some cases this hope was realized. However, funding cutbacks, inadequate resources, and denial by patients of the need for continued follow-up have limited the success of deinstitutionalization; in fact, 25–50% of discharged younger schizophrenic patients receive no outpatient treatment at all (2). Lacking financial resources and unable to function socially, many patients have ended up living on the streets or in cheap boarding homes, exploited by other denizens of the street and poorly cared for by the medical profession, until they decompensate sufficiently to require brief emergency treatment, after which they are returned to their previous situation. Solving the problem of homeless mental patients involves questions of how society is to pay for their care and whether their liberty is preferable to treatment that might be humane but against their wishes.

DEPRESSION

Twenty-five percent of patients recovering from an acute schizophrenic psychosis become depressed (3). Depression may be expressed in the context of schizophrenia as psychomotor retardation, deteriorated appearance, lack of energy, disinterest, anhedonia, emotional withdrawal, fatigue, and hopelessness. "Postpsychotic" depression usually lasts 4–12 months.

IMPAIRED CAPACITY FOR INFORMED CONSENT

To give informed consent, a patient must:

- understand the illness and the need for treatment
- understand the consequences of agreeing to or refusing therapy
- be provided with enough information about potential risks and benefits to be able to make a rational decision
- know about alternative therapies that other competent practitioners might recommend
- not be coerced (i.e., be threatened with such dire consequences that any reasonable person would be expected to accede).

Being psychotic is not incompatible with giving informed consent. However, if delusional or disorganized thinking impairs the patient's capacity to understand the ramifications of consenting to or refusing medical or psychiatric treatment, consent or refusal may not be valid. For example, the psychotic patient who denies being ill is not capable of truly understanding why treatment is needed or how it might help. Refusal of medication by a patient who believes that it is poisoned is not based on a rational appreciation of the treatment and is therefore not valid. Patients who agree to treatment out of a delusional belief that it will confer magical powers also are not making an informed decision, even if they are cooperative.

Once it has been determined that a patient cannot give informed consent or refusal, a decision about involuntary treatment must be made. In emergencies, a physician may institute treatment against a patient's wishes if the treatment is expected to preserve the life or health of the patient or other people. In non-emergent situations it usually is necessary for a court to make a legal decision based on information from the patient, the physician, and others about the patient's behalf in evaluating and deciding about the treatment. The capacity of all psychotic patients to understand and consent to treatment must be evaluated in order to prevent giving treatments without someone to protect their interest to patients whose consent is not truly informed, and in order to permit involuntary treatment when the potential benefits outweigh the harm of overriding the patient's wish not to be treated.

■ LABORATORY FINDINGS

Modern technology has made it possible to study disturbances in brain function in schizophrenia, particularly in the frontal and periventricular (i.e., near the limbic system) regions. Pneumoencephalography and computerized tomography (CT) of the head consistently reveal enlargement of the lateral and third ventricles and dilatation of cortical fissures and sulci in about 50% of schizophrenic patients (4). Patients with enlarged ventricles are more likely to have poor premorbid adjustment, negative symptoms, and evidence of intellectual impairment than are those with normal CT scans (5). Enlarged cerebral vertricles in schizophrenia do not seem to be a result of drug therapy, as the abnormality is present before the patient is ever treated; ventricular enlargement does not appear to be either progressive or reversible (6). Regional cerebral blood flow (rCBF) and positron emission tomography (PET) studies have been used to study metabolic activity in the cerebral cortex. Preliminary results of these studies suggest a deficiency in activation of a region of the frontal cortex (dorsolateral prefrontal cortex) in response to a demand for cognitive activity (7). There is no practical laboratory test for schizophrenia, and the principal application in clinical practice of laboratory testing is to rule out specific organic mental syndromes.

■ COURSE

Schizophrenia has traditionally been considered a chronic condition with isolated, withdrawn, and eccentric behavior prior to acute psychosis and progressive deterioration of functioning subsequently. Active symptoms tend to deteriorate over time, with positive symptoms being replaced with negative ones and organized delusions being replaced with disorganization (2). However, a number of chronic schizophrenic patients stabilize or even become more functional over time (8). The prognosis of schizophrenia is better if the patient rapidly becomes psychotic in response to an obvious precipitant, has reasonably good premorbid adjustment, exhibits confusion, affective symptoms, and positive symptoms, and has a family history of a mood disorder.

■ ETIOLOGY

Causes of psychotic cases of mania, depression, and organic mental syndromes are the same as the causes of the nonpsychotic varieties. Brief reactive psychoses probably are related to exaggeration of pathological defenses such as the tendency to keep apart ideas and emotions of opposite value (for example, being unable to conceive of loving and hating the same person) leading to extremely disorganized mental states under stress. Of the other functional psychoses, the most work has gone into studying the etiology of schizophrenia, which clearly has multifactorial causes.

BIOLOGICAL FACTORS

Family, twin, and adoptive studies provide powerful evidence that genetic factors predispose to the development of schizophrenia. However, although incomplete penetrance has been suggested, the exact mode of transmission is not known (9). Part of what is inherited may be a propensity to dysfunction in connections between the limbic system and regions of the frontal cortex that must synthesize complex emotional information. One result is inability to distinguish between relevant and irrelevant information, with resulting overreaction to unimportant information, inability to respond to significant input, and deficits in concept formation (10). This dysfunction may be derived from a disturbance in activity of the neurotransmitter dopamine and its receptors, at least in patients with positive symptoms (11). Disturbances in other neurotransmitters have not been demonstrated as consistently.

PSYCHOSOCIAL FACTORS

Psychological stresses do not cause schizophrenia. However, certain factors aggravate the disorder. Prominent among these are living in a setting in which the patient is made to feel guilty about not living up to unrealistic expectations, in which people are intrusive rather than supportive, in which communication is skewed, and in which discord, hostility, and intense emotions are expressed openly (12). The more time a patient spends in such an environment, the greater the risk of relapse (13).

■ DIFFERENTIAL DIAGNOSIS

It is common error to assume that any psychosis is functional. Organic mental syndromes, especially delirium, are much more likely to cause psychoses that are encountered in the general hospital or emergency room. Interictal states and partial complex seizures may produce confusion, mood swings, odd beliefs, extensive note taking, loquaciousness, and unusual religious and philosophical preoccupations. If a routine EEG is normal, a sleep-deprived EEG may reveal the abnormality. Stimulants, phencyclidine and withdrawal from alcohol can produce hallucinations, delusions, paranoia, and agitation. These syndromes (Chapter 6) usually resolve within hours to days, but stimulant psychoses may persist for months. There are also a number of functional psychiatric disorders that occasionally are associated with symptoms that are or appear to be psychotic. These are discussed below.

OBSESSIVE COMPULSIVE DISORDER

Obsessions are recurrent disturbing ideas that force themselves into the patient's mind despite attempts to resist them. Unlike delusions, these ideas are markedly different from the patient's usual thoughts, are not acted upon, and are recognized by the patient as abnormal and foreign. Bizarre compulsions may so disrupt everyday functioning as to mimic psychotic behavior.

MULTIPLE PERSONALITY

Multiple personality is a rare disorder in which different personalities or portions of personalities are dissociated (split off) from the main personality, taking full or partial control at various times. Patients with this condition may have auditory hallucinations that seem to be coming from within their heads and that represent communications from the other personalities. Since hallucinations imply loss of the ability to distinguish the real from the imaginary, these patients are by definition psychotic when they hear voices. Symptoms that distinguish multiple personality from schizophrenia include losing track of time, doing things the patient does not remember, finding objects the patient does not remember obtaining, finding notes in unfamiliar handwriting, and having periods of acting and speaking in unfamiliar manners. The mental experience of each personality is less fragmented than in schizophrenia, and the usual disruptions of thinking and logic are absent. Many patients with multiple personality disorder have an early history of physical and sexual abuse.

MALINGERING

In general medical practice, few patients fake psychotic symptoms, and those who do usually do so in an attempt to feel some control over an actual psychosis by convincing themselves that they are just pretending to be ill. Simulation of psychosis is much more common in the legal system. In most of these cases there is evidence of antisocial behavior that clearly predated the onset of the alleged psychosis and clearcut gain such as being found not guilty by reason of insanity. The malingerer usually appears psychotic only while being observed, different examiners obtain different histories and symptoms, and symptoms reflect the patient's idea of psychosis rather than typical symptoms. However, a few experienced malingerers are so adept at falsifying psychosis, and some truly psychotic patients engage in such blatant antisocial behavior, that only an expert can identify the bona fide patient.

FACTITIOUS DISORDER WITH PSYCHOLOGICAL SYMPTOMS

This is a rare form of conscious simulation of psychosis. Rather than feigning hallucinations, delusions, and incoherence for obvious gain, the goal of the patient with a factitious disorder appears to be considered psychotic. Like the malingerer, the patient has symptoms that vary with the examiner and that reflect an idea of psychosis rather than actual symptoms. The patient may have had multiple hospitalizations under different names.

GANSER'S SYNDROME

Ganser's syndrome is an uncommon form of unconscious simulation of psychosis in which the patient acts in a silly or impossible manner and gives "approximate" answers on mental status testing. For example, when asked to add 2 and 2, the patient may answer "5," or when asked "who is buried in Grant's Tomb?" replies, "Lincoln." Ganser's syndrome is often associated with dissociative symptoms such as amnesia, disorientation, perceptual distortions, and fugue.

■ TREATMENT

Some aspects of all psychoses have a common treatment. Specific disorders require additional therapies, the most important of which are addressed below.

DRUG THERAPY OF PSYCHOSIS

Antipsychotic drugs (neuroleptics) are used to treat all psychoses except those caused by withdrawal from CNS depressants. The potency of these medications in ameliorating psychosis and producing neurological side effects parallels their potency in blocking dopamine receptors in the brain. Calcium channel blockade may be an additional mechanism for some preparations.

PREPARATIONS AND DOSAGE

Five classes of antipsychotic agents are now available in the United States: phenothiazines, thioxanthenes, butyrophenones, indolones, and dibenzoxazepines. Depot injectable preparations of fluphenazine and haloperidol are used to treat noncompliant chronic schizophrenic patients. Schizophrenic patients with predominantly negative symptoms have been treated with the experimental diphenyl butylpiperidine neuroleptics, pimozide and penfluridol. Neuroleptics differ mainly in their anticholinergic properties and their tendency to produce sedation, hypotension, and acute extrapyramidal reactions. Usual doses and side effects are summarized in Table 3.

There are a number of metabolic pathways for antipsychotic drugs (14). Chlorpromazine and thioridazine have many active metabolites, whereas haloperidol and thioridazine are metabolized only to inactive compounds. Parenteral administration avoids initial metabolism by the liver, making the availability of the neuroleptic four to ten times greater than it is after oral administration. Some low-potency neuroleptics such as chlorpromazine and thioridazine induce their own metabolism after a few weeks of treatment, so that blood levels decrease (15). The half-life of all neuroleptics is long (20–40 hours), and metabolites are detected in the urine months after the drug is discontinued. This probably explains why recurrence of psychosis is delayed after medication is discontinued.

SIDE EFFECTS AND INTERACTIONS

Postural hypotension and sedation are common problems with low potency neuroleptics (i.e., neuroleptics that require higher doses to produce a given effect such as chlorpromazine, thioridazine, and chlorprothixene). Low potency drugs also lower

TABLE 3. Antipsychotic Drugs (Neuroleptics) Available in the United States

Class and Drug	Trade Name	Usual Daily Oral Dose (mg)	Usual Single I.M. Dose (mg)	Sedative Properties	Anticholinergic Properties	Hypotensive Effects	Parkinsonian Effects
Phenothiazines							
Chlorpromazine	Thorazine	300–800	25–50	Very high	High	Moderate–high	Moderate
Trifluopromazine	Vesprin	100–150	20–60	Moderate	Moderate	Moderate	High
Thioridazine	Mellaril	200–700	—	High	Very high	Moderate–high	Low
Mesoridazine	Serentil	75–300	25	High	Moderate–high	Moderate	Low
Acetophenazine	Tindal	60–120	—	Moderate	Moderate	Low	Moderate
Perphenazine	Trilafon	8–40	5–10	Moderate	Moderate–low	Low–moderate	Moderate–high
Trifluoperazine	Stelazine	6–20	1–2	Low	Low	Low	High
Fluphenazine	Prolixin	1–20	12.5–5.0 [a]	Low	Low	Low	High
Thioxanthenes							
Chlorprothixene	Taractan	50–400	25–50	High		Moderate	Moderate
Thiothixene	Navane	6–30	2–4	Low–moderate	Low	Moderate	Moderate–high
Butyrophenones							
Haloperidol	Haldol	6–20	2–5 [b]	Low	Very low	Very low	Very high
Dibenzoxazepines							
Loxapine	Loxitane	60–100	12.5–50	Low–moderate	Moderate	Low	Moderate
Dihydroindolones							
Molindone	Moban	50–100	—	Low–moderate	Moderate	Very low	Low–moderate

[a] 1.25–2.5 cc of depot form every 1–3 weeks for maintenance
[b] 1–4 cc of depot form every 4 weeks for maintenance

the seizure threshold and produce more anticholinergic side effects such as constipation, dry mouth, blurred vision, and tachycardia. All antipsychotic drugs can produce weight gain, easy sunburning (photosensitivity), and, rarely, leukopenia and agranulocytosis. At doses greater than 800 mg/day, thioridazine causes irreversible pigmentary retinopathy.

Neuroleptics produce a number of acute extrapyramidal syndromes (EPS), common examples of which are summarized in Table 4 (15–17). Some clinicians recommend adding antiparkinsonian drugs (e.g., 1–4 mg/day of benztropine or 2–4 mg/day of biperiden) when neuroleptics are started to prevent dystonia and parkinsonism and enhance compliance. Others advise that extrapyramidal symptoms are rare when the dosage of the neuroleptic is adjusted carefully (17). Prophylactic antiparkinsonian therapy often is not necessary with low potency neuroleptics, but it is definitely indicated for patients with a past history of acute dystonia with neuroleptics and for adolescent and young adult males receiving high potency neuroleptics such as haloperidol, trifluoperazine, or fluphenazine (17). Since the duration of action of neuroleptics is much longer than that of antiparkinsonian drugs, extrapyramidal side effects may re-emerge when both medications are discontinued at the same time.

The two most serious complications of neuroleptics are neuroleptic malignant syndrome, which can appear at any time in the course of treatment, and tardive dyskinesia, which usually begins after long-term administration but may appear after only six months. Patients should be warned about these syndromes, the characteristics and management of which are summarized in Table 5 (18). Clozapine, an experimental neuroleptic that may soon be available on a limited basis in the United States, does not appear to cause tardive dyskinesia and may improve it. Clozapine also may be more useful than other antipsychotic drugs for schizophrenia with prominent negative symptoms. However it has a 1% incidence of potentially fatal bone marrow suppression.

Sedating neuroleptics such as chlorpromazine potentiate other CNS depressants, and anticholinergic effects are additive with other anticholinergic drugs. Antiparkinsonian drugs, carbamazepine, phenobarbital, and phenytoin enhance metabolism of neuroleptics, decreasing serum concentrations and sometimes the clinical effectiveness of the antipsychotic (15). The

TABLE 4. **Acute Neuroleptic-Induced Extrapyramidal Syndromes (EPS)**

Syndrome	Incidence	Onset	Manifestations	Predisposing Factors	Prevention	Treatment
Akathisia	25–50%	First week, often after first dose	Inner restlessness Inability to sit still Diaphoresis May be mistaken for agitation	High potency neuroleptic	Use lower doses	Reduce dose of neuroleptic Beta blockers Clonidine Lorazepam Anticholinergics not effective
Dystonia	2–50%	First 1–3 days	Torticollis Opisthotonos Oculogyric crisis Grimacing May be mistaken for mannerisms	High potency neuroleptic	Use low potency neuroleptic Prophylactic antiparkinsonism drug	Parenteral antiparkinsonian or antihistamine (e.g., diphenhydramine)
Parkinsonism	Up to 90%	Within one month	Akinesia Mask-like face Rigidity Tremor Shuffling, stooped gait May be mistaken for withdrawal, blunted affect, or decreased spontaneity	Long-acting drugs; Parenteral administration High dose Young male Past history of EPS	Prophylactic antiparkinsonian Low dose Use low potency drugs	Anticholinergics Amantadine

TABLE 5. **Tardive Dyskinesia and Neuroleptic Malignant Syndrome**

Syndrome	Incidence	Peak Onset	Risk Factors	Manifestations	Treatment	Prevention
Tardive Dyskinesia	10–45%	6–24 months or later	Older female Brain damage Mood disorder Large total amount of neuroleptic taken	Choreoathetosis and dystonia of tongue, lips, extremities, trunk, and sometimes respiratory muscles	Discontinue drug (improvement may take 3 yrs or more) Experimental treatments: calcium antagonists, propranolol, clonidine, reserpine, deanol, lecithin, -vinyl GABA, clonazepam	Use lowest possible dose "Drug holidays" not proven helpful Use alternative to neuroleptic
Neuroleptic Malignant Syndrome	0.5–1%	Immediate or delayed	Intramuscular administration High potency neuroleptics Male, younger than 40 Alcoholism Delilitation Neurological or medical illness Psychosis other than schizophrenia	Hyperthermia Extrapyramidal syndromes Rigidity Myoglobinuria Renal failure Autonomic instability Delirium Catatonia Elevated WBC, CBK, and urinary myoglobin	Cooling, hydration, bromocriptine, dantrolene, amantadine, calcium channel blockers Sometimes subsides spontaneously, but mortality = 4–30%	Use alternative to neuroleptic

combination of carbamazepine and neuroleptics can produce delirium. Lithium added to high potency neuroleptics such as haloperidol may produce severe extrapyramidal syndromes, delirium, and ataxia that on occasion have been reported to be irreversible (19). Neuroleptics raise antidepressant blood levels by as much as 50%.

USE OF NEUROLEPTICS

Neuroleptics can be prescribed for a variety of psychoses according to these guidelines (18, 20–22):

1. Start a neuroleptic as early as possible in the course of acute schizophrenia. Rapid treatment leads to more rapid remission, and early resolution of the first episode may decrease vulnerability to subsequent decompensation.

2. Use the lowest effective dose. High doses of neuroleptics increase the risk of tardive dyskinesia and produce acute side effects that reduce compliance and mimic psychotic symptoms (Table 4). Higher doses are sometimes necessary for severely psychotic patients, but most acute schizophrenic patients respond to 300 mg/day of chlorpromazine or its equivalent, and many can be maintained on much lower doses (e.g., 25–75 mg/day). Agitated delirious and demented patients usually require very low doses of nonsedating neuroleptics (Chapter 5). Some psychotically depressed patients may need higher doses of neuroleptics than schizophrenic patients.

3. Offer the medication orally. Many psychotic patients agree to take a neuroleptic if they have an opportunity to think about it, feel some control over the treatment, and are reassured that side effects will be treated promptly. If a patient in need of an antipsychotic continues to refuse necessary treatment, a neuroleptic can be given intramuscularly if principles of involuntary treatment are followed. Neurological and hypotensive side effects are more common with intramuscular dosage.

4. Avoid frequent or high dose intramuscular administration for agitation. "Rapid neuroleptization," in which multiple intramuscular doses are administered to combative patients until they are sedated, is no more effective than standard oral dosing and is more likely to cause extrapyramidal reactions.

5. Treat severely violent behavior with intravenous haloper-

idol and/or lorazepam. Intravenous haloperidol with or without lorazepam is probably the safest and most effective treatment for severe agitation and psychosis of any etiology except CNS depressant withdrawal. After a 5 mg test dose, 5–10 mg boluses of haloperidol are used as frequently as necessary; single injections as high as 75 mg and total daily doses of 530 mg have been given safely. Alternatively, a mixture or 3–10 mg of haloperidol and 1–10 mg of lorazepam mixed in the same syringe may be administered intravenously. Sedating neuroleptics and tranquilizers may make paranoid patients more agitated because these drugs interfere with hypervigilance that the patients feel is necessary to protect them from danger.

6. *Give a neuroleptic to which the patient or a family member has responded.* Familial patterns of metabolism predict a better response to medications that have been of benefit to a blood relative.

7. *Continue the neuroleptic for at least one year after the first episode of acute schizophrenia.* An attempt can then be made to withdraw the medication very gradually, but the previous dose should be reinstituted at the first indication of relapse. Group, family, and occupational therapy reduce the need for medication. Reliable patients may be able to avoid continuous drug therapy if they can be followed closely and treated rapidly whenever psychotic symptoms begin to re-emerge.

8. *Always think about noncompliance.* The most common cause of relapse is discontinuation of the medication because the patient does not like the side effects, denies being sick enough to need any more treatment, or prefers psychotic symptoms to the rigors of reality. Patients should be repeatedly questioned as to their feelings about and compliance with neuroleptics.

9. *Consider alternatives or adjuncts to neuroleptics for patients with tardive dyskinesia or a history of neuroleptic malignant syndrome.* Lorazepam alone may reduce the amount of neuroleptic needed and sometimes sufficiently tranquilizes agitated psychotic patients. Reserpine may have additive antipsychotic actions with neuroleptics and has the additional advantage of ameliorating tardive dyskinesia in some patients. Short-acting barbiturates such as amobarbital can be used for emergency tranquilization in patients without organic brain disease, prophyria, or increased intracranial pressure. Verapamil, baclofen, droperidol,

and L-tryptophan also have been used occasionally as antipsychotic agents.

10. Withdraw the medication if it is not helping. Some patients simply do not benefit from neuroleptics. If the patient is no worse without the medication, the risks of continued treatment do not justify the meager benefits.

PSYCHOLOGICAL AND BEHAVIORAL MANAGEMENT OF PSYCHOSIS

Different measures are employed for treating acute and chronic psychoses. The following are the most important goals in *acute* treatment.

REASSURE THE PATIENT

Psychotic patients become agitated because they feel threatened. Reassurance that they are safe and that the physician is in control can de-escalate potentially dangerous behavior.

ENSURE THE SAFETY OF PATIENT AND PHYSICIAN

It is impossible to reassure a patient if either the patient or the doctor is in danger from the patient's behavior. Guaranteeing that the treatment setting is safe involves several precautions:

- *Do not sit too close to the patient.* Psychotic patients have increased "body space." Excessive physical closeness makes the patient feel more threatened and therefore more threatening, and also places the doctor within striking range.
- *Have assistance available.* If a sufficient number of skilled personnel who can control the patient's behavior are available, the patient is less likely to need them. However, if the patient feels that the environment is not safe, he may test the doctor's ability to provide the necessary controls.
- *Allow an escape route for patient and physician.* Leaving the door open and sitting near the door makes it easier to get away if the patient becomes threatening. Any potentially dangerous patient who wishes to leave an interview or examination should be allowed to do so. The police can be called once the patient is out of the room.
- *Pay attention to feelings about the patient.* Whenever the doc-

tor feels unaccountably afraid in the presence of a superficially calm patient, the patient may be nonverbally communicating impending loss of control. Any feeling that the patient could be dangerous should be taken seriously.

- *Never see a patient who has a weapon.* A surprising number of patients are armed when they come to the emergency room or hospital. These patients should be disarmed immediately by trained personnel.

BE PREPARED TO RESTRAIN THE PATIENT

Acutely agitated patients whose behavior cannot be controlled with reassurance and medication may need to be physically restrained. Safe restraint involves:

- *Training of all personnel.* A protocol for restraint should be practiced by all concerned.
- *Sufficient numbers.* It takes at least five people to restrain a patient safely: one for each limb and one to coordinate the procedure. A sufficient show of force may convince the patient to cooperate with the procedure, while insufficient numbers may be so frightening or insulting that the patient feels compelled to struggle.
- *Neutrality of the physician.* Physicians and students should not participate in the physical process of restraint because they are not trained in the procedure and because they will lose the neutrality and objectivity that are necessary to a productive doctor–patient relationship.
- *Close observation.* Physically restrained patients may aspirate, strangle, or develop myoglobinuria from prolonged struggling.

ADDRESS PSYCHOSOCIAL CRISES

Exacerbations of chronic psychoses often are associated with a stress, trauma, expectation, or loss in the family or residence in which the patient lives. Controlling the environmental problem decreases the need for psychotic coping mechanisms. It may be necessary to find a new living situation if the people with whom the patient resides continue to encourage psychotic behavior.

REDUCE PHYSICAL STRESSORS

Illnesses, many medications, alcohol, and illicit drugs increase confusion and weaken the patient's defenses.

FIND OUT WHAT HAS BEEN HELPFUL IN THE PAST

If a family member, friend, co-worker, or teacher has helped the patient to reorganize in the past, that person should be involved in the current treatment. The patient should be encouraged to recommence activities that have been useful before, such as exercising, reading, or attending group meetings.

HAVE THE OUTPATIENT TEAM VISIT THE PATIENT IN THE HOSPITAL

This will increase the likelihood of the patient's following through with outpatient treatment. The patient should have a follow-up appointment at discharge.

The focus of treatment shifts for *chronically* psychotic patients, most of whom are schizophrenic. The primary goals in this setting are to:

INVOLVE THE FAMILY

Many families want to participate in the patient's treatment but do not know how to help. Interventions that are particularly helpful include:

- *Education.* The patient and the family should be taught about factors that increase and relieve psychotic symptoms.
- *Relief of guilt.* Information about biological causes of mania and schizophrenia makes it easier for families not to blame themselves for the patient's illness. Inappropriate guilt leads to overprotectiveness, intrusiveness, or avoidance of the patient.
- *Modulation of emotion.* Environments in which intense and conflicting emotions are openly expressed aggravate schizophrenia. The family should be helped to control and deal constructively with anger and interpersonal disputes. Inability to tolerate and work through loss are often important problems in the families of patients with mania and psychotic depression.
- *Developing realistic expectations.* Unrealistic expectations

that the patient perform beyond his or her capabilities induce strongly mixed feelings that call forth psychotic defenses. Without giving up on the patient, the family should learn to adopt realistic goals. For example, the patient may not be able to work as an executive, but may be able to hold regular employment in a stockroom.

PROVIDE AN ONGOING RELATIONSHIP

Patients who are prone to chronic or recurrent psychoses may not need to be seen too frequently, but they should be monitored at regular intervals. A brief (15-minute) visit is sufficient to reassure the patient of the doctor's availability and provide a stable social contact for a patient who may not have many other meaningful interactions. The patient should be called if one appointment is missed without notice or if several appointments are missed after notifying the doctor, since missed appointments may be the first sign of impending decompensation.

AVOID EXCESSIVE INTIMACY

Schizophrenic and paranoid patients are threatened by attempts to get too close to them emotionally and are reassured by appropriate professional distance.

PROVIDE SUPPORT AND ADVICE

If the physician is a "real" person psychotic fantasies and impulses are not encouraged.

AVOID AGGRESSIVE ATTEMPTS AT INSIGHT

Individual psychotherapy early after remission of an acute schizophrenic psychosis often makes the patient worse; it is more likely to be helpful later on. Discussions with the patient should focus on everyday problems while avoiding exploration of unconscious motivations that feel overwhelming to the patient.

TEACH SOCIAL AND OCCUPATIONAL SKILLS

Groups, sheltered workshops, social skills training, and related therapies help chronically psychotic patients to strengthen abilities that are impaired by the illness.

WORK WITH SOCIAL AGENCIES

Many chronically psychotic patients are involved with multiple social agencies such as mental health centers, halfway houses, welfare, and medicaid. The physician is often in the best position to coordinate the activities of these agencies.

TREAT SUBSTANCE ABUSE

Illicit drugs and alcohol aggravate psychoses and may reduce blood levels of neuroleptics. Aggressive treatment is essential to control of the psychosis.

■ REFERENCES

1. Andreasen NC: Negative symptoms in schizophrenia. Arch Gen Psychiatry 1982; 39:784–794
2. Pfohl B, Andreasen NC: Schizophrenia: diagnosis and classification, in Psychiatry Update: The American Psychiatric Association Annual Review, vol. 5. Edited by Frances AJ, Hales RE. Washington DC, American Psychiatric Press, 1986
3. McGlashan TH: Postpsychotic depression in schizophrenia. Arch Gen Psychiatry 1976; 33:231–239
4. Weinberger DF, Torrey EF: Lateral cerebral ventricular enlargement in chronic schizophrenia. Arch Gen Psychiatry 1979; 36:935–939
5. Crow TJ: Molecular pathology of schizophrenia: more than one disease process? Br Med J 1980; 260:66–68
6. Weinberger DR: CAT scan findings in schizophrenia: speculation on the meaning of it all. J Psychiatr Res 1984; 18:477–490
7. Weinberger DR, Kleinman JE: Observations on the brain in schizophrenia, in Psychiatry Update: The American Psychiatric Association Annual Review, vol. 5. Edited by Frances AJ, Hales RE. Washington DC, American Psychiatric Press, 1986
8. Shapiro S, Skinner EA, Kessler LG, et al: Utilization of health and mental health services. Arch Gen Psychiatry 1984; 41:971–978
9. Risch N, Baron M: Segregation analysis of schizophrenia and related disorders. Am J Hum Genet 1984; 36:1039–1059
10. Nuechterlein KH, Dawson ME: Vulnerability and stress factors in the developmental course of schizophrenic disorders. Schizophr Bull 1984; 10:158–159
11. Lee T, Seeman P, Tourtellotte WW, et al: Binding of 3H-neuroleptics and 3H-apomorphine in schizophrenic brains. Nature 1978; 274:897–900
12. Leff J, Vaughn C: The role of maintenance therapy and relatives'

expressed emotion in relapse of schizophrenia: a two-year follow-up. Br J Psychiatry 1981; 139:102–104

13. Brown GW: Influence of family life on the course of schizophrenia: a replication. Br Psychiatry 1972; 121: 241–258

14. Ko GN, Korpi ER, Linnoila M: On the clinical relevance and methods of quantification of plasma concentrations of neuroleptics. J Clin Psychopharmacol 1985; 5:344–347

15. Baldessarini RJ: Drugs and the treatment of psychiatric disorders, in The Pharmacological Basis of Therapeutics. Edited by Gilman AG, Goodman LS, Rall TW, et al. New York, Macmillan, 1985

16. Greenhill MH, Gralinck A (Eds): Psychopharmacology and Psychotherapy. New York, Free Press, 1982

17. Ayd F: Prophylactic antiparkinsonian drug therapy: pros and cons. International Drug Therapy Newsletter 1986; 121:5–6

18. Dubovsky SL, Ringel SP: Psychopharmacologic treatment in neurology. Journal of Neurologic Rehabilitation 1987; 1:51–66

19. Izzo KL, Brody R: Rehabilitation in lithium toxicity. Arch Phys Med Rehabil 1985; 66:779–782

20. Davis JM, Andriukaitis S: The natural course of schizophrenia and effective maintenance drug treatment. J Clin Psychopharmacol 1986; 6:25–105

21. Tesar GE, Murray GB, Cassem NH: Use of high-dose intravenous haloperidol in the treatment of agitated cardiac patients. J Clin Psychopharmacol 1985; 5:344–347

22. Adams F, Fernandez F, Anderson BE: Emergency pharmacotherapy of delirium in the critically ill cancer patient. Psychosomatics 1986; 27(suppl):33–37

INDEX

Abstinence syndromes, 141, 146-147
Alcohol abuse
  drug therapy, 159
  incidence, 138
  insomnia and, 84-85
  physical complications, 148
  withdrawal syndrome, 144
  See also Substance abuse
Alexithymia, 98
All-or-nothing thinking, 20
Anxiety
  associated problems, 57-59
  categories, 51-52
  compared with fear, 50
  course, 60
  differential diagnosis, 62-64
  etiology, 60-62
  family history, 56-57
  incidence, 49-50
  laboratory findings, 59-60
  management, 71-75
  past history, 56
  in patients with organic mental syndromes, 134
  present illness, 55-56
  resistance to treatment, 75-76
  signs and symptoms, 50-51
  somatoform disorders and, 107
  treatment, 64-71
Aprosodias, 16-17

Bright light therapy, 43
Briquet's syndrome, 100

Cocaine abuse, 138, 149, 160
Cyclothymia, 16

Delirium
  course, 126-127

Delirium *(cont)*
  depression and, 23
  etiology, 127-128
  signs and symptoms, 121
  See also Organic mental syndromes
Dementia
  course, 126-127
  depression and, 23-24
  described, 121
  etiology, 127-128
  subtle presentations, 126
  See also Organic mental syndromes
Depression
  anxiety and, 57
  associated problems, 8-12
  categories, 4-6
  course, 17
  differential diagnosis, 21-27
  etiology, 17-21
  family history, 8
  incidence, 1
  laboratory findings, 12-14
  nonpharmacologic treatments, 43-44
  past history, 7
  in patients with organic mental syndromes, 135
  present illness, 6-7
  in schizophrenic patients, 174
  signs and symptoms, 1-4
  somatoform disorders and, 106-107
  subtle presentations, 14-17
  talking to depressed patients, 44-47
  treatment, 27-43
Dissociative disorders, 130
Drug therapy
  alcoholism, 159
  anxiety, 65-71
  depression, 29-43
  insomnia, 92-94
  organic mental syndromes, 134-136
  psychosis, 180-187
  sleep disorders, 94-95
  somatoform disorders, 109-111
  substance abuse disorders, 159-160
Dysthymia, 5, 15-16

Electroconvulsive therapy (ECT), 37-38

Ganser's syndrome, 179
Grief, 6, 19, 25-26

Homelessness, 171-174
Hypersomnias, 78, 80
Hypochondriasis, 58, 100

Informed consent, 174-175
Insomnia, 78, 79, 92-94, 134-135
    See also Sleep disorders
Intoxication syndromes, 141, 142

Learned helplessness, 21

Malingering, 90, 108, 178-179
Mania, 9, 16, 23
Manic depressive illness, 5-6, 16
Marijuana, 149
Mental status examination (MSE), 114-117
Mitral valve prolapse (MVP), 59
Multiple personality disorder, 178
Munchausen's syndrome, 108, 179

Narcolepsy, 80
Narcotics abuse, 148, 160

Obsessive compulsive disorder, 52-53, 178
Organic mental syndromes
    anxiety and, 62-64
    associated problems, 123-124
    categories, 120-122
    course, 126-127

Organic mental syndromes *(cont)*
    diagnosis, 114-117
    differential diagnosis, 128-130
    etiology, 127-128
    family history, 123
    laboratory findings, 124-126
    management, 132-133
    past history, 123
    present illness, 122-123
    signs and symptoms, 117-120
    somatoform disorders and, 107
    treatment, 130-136

Panic disorder, 52, 65
Paranoia, 169-170
Parasomnias, 79, 82
Personality disorders, 130
Phobias, 53, 66
Physicians, addiction in, 161-162
Posttraumatic stress disorder (PTSD), 53-54, 66
Psychoactive substance abuse, 139-140
Psychoactive substance dependence, 138-139
Psychosis
    anxiety and, 64
    associated problems, 171-175
    categories, 167-170
    course, 176
    differential diagnosis, 177-179
    etiology, 176-177
    history, 170-171
    laboratory findings, 175-176
    management, 187-191
    signs and symptoms, 164-166
    treatment, 179-191

Schizophrenia, 26-27, 108, 129, 167-169
Seasonal affective disorder (SADs), 6
Sedative abuse, 148
Self-fulfilling prophecies, 20
Sleep deprivation therapy, 43-44